Surgical Atlas of Cerebral Revascularization

Ying Mao • Wei Zhu • Jianping Song
Editors

Surgical Atlas of Cerebral Revascularization

Springer

Editors
Ying Mao
Department of Neurosurgery
Huashan Hospital, Shanghai Medical College, Fudan University
Shanghai
China

Wei Zhu
Department of Neurosurgery
Huashan Hospital, Shanghai Medical College, Fudan University
Shanghai
China

Jianping Song
Department of Neurosurgery
Huashan Hospital, Shanghai Medical College, Fudan University
Shanghai
China

ISBN 978-981-16-0373-0 ISBN 978-981-16-0374-7 (eBook)
https://doi.org/10.1007/978-981-16-0374-7

This Springer imprint is published by the registered company Springer Nature Singapore Pte Ltd.
The registered company address is: 152 Beach Road, #21-01/04 Gateway East, Singapore 189721, Singapore

Preface

We aim to summarize the current surgical strategies for cerebral revascularization in the treatment of complex neurovascular diseases based on a single-center experience over the last 30 years. Complex intracranial (IC) aneurysms are mostly large/giant and irregular and do not have enough collateral compensation, so they are difficult to directly clip or embolize, leading to a high fatality rate of 68–85%. We have established the extracranial-intracranial (EC-IC) bypass strategy based on our clinical experience. For complex IC carotid artery aneurysms, the types of EC-IC bypass are determined based on preoperative hemodynamic evaluations. For complex middle cerebral artery (MCA) aneurysms, the types of EC-IC bypass are determined based on angioarchitecture. Furthermore, various IC-IC bypasses have been introduced into our surgical arsenal, with the advantages of not requiring graft vessel harvesting and preferable matching of donor and recipient arteries. The favorable outcome rate of complex IC aneurysm after cerebral revascularization remained ≥85–90%. In addition, the unique superficial temporal artery to MCA (STA-MCA) bypass (single or double) procedure combined with encephalo-duro-myo-synangiosis (EDMS) for Moyamoya disease has been successfully utilized in over 10,000 cases in our hospital. We believe that the cerebral revascularization technique is a basic and indispensable skill for neurosurgeons.

Shanghai, China

Ying Mao
Wei Zhu
Jianping Song

Introduction

The treatment of giant aneurysms has always been a challenge in the field of neurovascular disease. Giant aneurysms are not only larger in size but are also associated with thrombosis development and calcification of the aneurysmal wall and neck, which often interfere with direct clipping. Most giant aneurysms have a wide neck with incomplete thrombus, making complete embolization almost impossible. Giant aneurysms at different sites have completely different hemodynamic characteristics. Moreover, aneurysms at the same site may exhibit very different hemodynamics among different individuals. Therefore, a careful assessment of each case is required before and during treatment to develop an individualized treatment plan.

Endovascular treatments and surgery are still the primary treatment approaches for giant aneurysms. The former includes occlusion of the parent artery, embolization of the aneurysm (including coiling and Onyx application), and stent- and balloon-assisted embolization of the aneurysm. Occlusion of the parent artery may completely occlude the aneurysm but can only be performed after careful assessment of cerebral hemodynamic and metabolic compensatory capacity. Stent- and balloon-assisted embolization techniques improve the success rate of complete aneurysmal neck embolization, but the elevated long-term recurrence rate of aneurysms is indisputable. Some patients may successfully undergo aneurysm trapping and reconstructive aneurysm clipping via craniotomy. However, in most patients, the hemodynamic and morphological features of the aneurysms make direct clipping impossible. Therefore, vascular reconstruction has become an indispensable and important approach in the treatment of giant intracranial aneurysms.

When treating giant internal carotid artery (ICA) aneurysms, the vascular reconstruction technique mainly refers to extracranial-intracranial bypass (EC-IC bypass), which includes high-flow (external carotid artery-radial artery-middle cerebral artery, ECA-RA-MCA, or external carotid artery-saphenous vein-middle cerebral artery, ECA-SV-MCA) and medium-flow (superficial temporal artery-radial artery-middle cerebral artery, STA-RA-MCA) bypass. Most researchers do not recommend the use of low-flow (STA-MCA) bypass. The preoperative hemodynamic assessment determines the selection of a bypass procedure with an appropriate flow rate. The assessment methods include the balloon occlusion test (BOT), the pressure drop test, single-photon emission computed tomography (SPECT), positron emission tomography (PET), computed tomography perfusion imaging (CTP), and xenon-enhanced CT (xenon-CT). Currently, there is not a single well-accepted test to accurately predict the tolerance of patients to permanent occlusion of the ICA. However, based on current clinical data, many centers have reported their own assessment methods for testing ICA occlusion tolerance, including BOT+PET, BOT+SPECT, and BOT+xenon-CT. We suggest using the "BOT+CTP" plan, which is simple, effective, and cost-efficient.

For MCA aneurysms, the hemodynamic differences are significant among giant aneurysms located in different MCA segments, and the treatment strategy should be adjusted accordingly. M1 aneurysms that involve important perforating branches such as lenticulostriate arteries cannot be directly clipped. In the case of a patient with a selectively positive BOT (BOT in the M1 segment), a medium- or high-flow EC-IC bypass (ECA-RA-MCA or STA-RA-MCA) can be combined with ipsilateral chronic ICA occlusion as treatment. The gradual decrease in intra-aneurysm blood flow is beneficial for establishing collateral lenticulostriate artery circulation and promoting ischemic tolerance in the supply area. Due to early thrombosis development in the giant aneurysm and the gradual decrease in intra-aneurysm blood flow, complete thrombosis of the aneurysm can be achieved in most cases. Moderate-flow (STA-RA-M3) bypass and trapping of the aneurysmal parent arteries can be used to treat aneurysms in the M2 segment (including the M2 bifurcation). Trapping of the aneurysmal parent arteries can be directly performed in most giant aneurysms beyond the M3 segment. However, cerebral ischemia may be present if the parent artery is the central artery or the artery of the angular gyrus. If necessary, aneurysm trapping should be performed after vascular reconstruction. In particular, intraoperative electrophysiological monitoring (including for motor evoked potentials, MEPs, and somatosensory evoked potentials, SEPs) plays an important role in assessing the tolerance to vascular occlusion and the timely identification of motor dysfunction due to various causes. Such monitoring is an essential safeguard for MCA aneurysm procedures. In addition, due to the variety of angioarchitectures and morphologies of MCA aneurysms and the large number of accompanying arteries, more rapid, minimally invasive, flexible IC-IC bypass is used. Extensive treatment approaches require further improvements in the microsurgical skills of neurosurgeons.

Most anterior communicating artery aneurysms can be directly or reconstructively clipped through the aneurysm body or neck. Vascular reconstruction is mainly used in cases in which A2 occlusion is required, including side-to-side A2-A2 or A3-A3 anastomoses in most cases.

Vascular reconstruction techniques applied for the treatment of aneurysms in the posterior circulation include EC-IC and IC-IC bypass. The main pattern is occipital artery-posterior inferior cerebellar artery (OA-PICA) bypass or superficial temporal artery-posterior cerebral artery (STA-PCA) bypass. Sometimes, due to the variable position and morphology of the posterior circulation aneurysm, it is necessary to use IC-IC bypass during surgery depending upon individual conditions. Sanai and his colleagues classified IC-IC bypass into four types to meet the requirements of vascular reconstruction in various situations: in situ bypass, reimplantation, reanastomosis, and IC bypass with graft. A high degree of surgical skills is required for these procedures because the operating sites of the posterior circulation aneurysm are close to important tissues and the operating space is limited. In addition, because of the generally poor tolerance to posterior circulation occlusion and the lack of accurate pre- and intraoperative assessment methods, a rapid bypass speed and high degree of technical skills are required for these procedures.

Although vascular reconstruction techniques have been widely used in the surgical treatment of complex IC aneurysms, further improvements to these techniques are still needed. The most common problem is how to evaluate the blood flow volume of the reconstructed vessels, including the blood flow volume of the blood vessels associated with the parent artery before and after occlusion as well as the reconstructed vessels. This information is key for correctly choosing a vascular reconstruction technique and for ensuring the effectiveness of treatment. Amin-Hanjani and his colleagues used magnetic resonance imaging noninvasive optimal vessel analysis (NOVA) to examine the flow rate of the blood vessels used in vascular reconstruction before surgery and to directly measure the flow rate during surgery. This method helps to obtain the required flow volume of the reconstructed vessel. Ultimately, the type of vascular reconstruction can be determined based on these measured flow rates. However, changes in blood flow after IC arterial occlusion are based on changes in the overall hemodynamics of the vascular network rather than the flow of a single artery. Thus, it is still necessary to perform brain metabolism assessments and functional measurements. The evaluation scheme needs to be further improved in future research.

The development of IC vascular reconstruction techniques began in 1969 when Yasargil first reported STA-MCA bypass. After several decades of development, this technique has been used to cure many complicated IC aneurysms that were previously incurable. However, the advancement of medical technology is endless. As people pay more attention to quality of life, more advanced vascular reconstruction techniques that are minimally invasive, rapid, and effective are needed to treat aneurysms. Thus, highly technical microsurgery skills are required. Lawton and his colleagues suggested that, in the future, vascular reconstruction for the treatment of IC aneurysms will focus on IC-IC bypass and even proposed that the "IC-IC bypass era" is coming. Such expectations require that our country's neurosurgeons not be satisfied with the current techniques but constantly improve upon existing treatment strategies and skills to benefit additional domestic patients.

Ying Mao
Department of Neurosurgery
Huashan Hospital, Shanghai Medical College, Fudan University
Shanghai, China

Contents

Editors and Contributors

Editors

Ying Mao, MD, PhD Huashan Hospital, Shanghai Medical College, Fudan University, Shanghai, China

Wei Zhu, MD, PhD Huashan Hospital, Shanghai Medical College, Fudan University, Shanghai, China

Jianping Song, MD, PhD Huashan Hospital, Shanghai Medical College, Fudan University, Shanghai, China

Contributors

Qingzhu An, MD, PhD Huashan Hospital, Shanghai Medical College, Fudan University, Shanghai, China

Liang Chen, MD, PhD Huashan Hospital, Shanghai Medical College, Fudan University, Shanghai, China

Yuxiang Gu, MD, PhD Huashan Hospital, Shanghai Medical College, Fudan University, Shanghai, China

Yu Lei, MD Huashan Hospital, Shanghai Medical College, Fudan University, Shanghai, China

Yujun Liao, MD Huashan Hospital, Shanghai Medical College, Fudan University, Shanghai, China

Peiliang Li, MD, PhD Huashan Hospital, Shanghai Medical College, Fudan University, Shanghai, China

Wei Ni, MD, PhD Huashan Hospital, Shanghai Medical College, Fudan University, Shanghai, China

Yi Qian, PhD Macquarie University, Sydney, Australia

Kai Quan, MD, PhD Huashan Hospital, Shanghai Medical College, Fudan University, Shanghai, China

Xiaowen Wang, MD, PhD Huashan Hospital, Shanghai Medical College, Fudan University, Shanghai, China

Bin Xu, MD, PhD Huashan Hospital, Shanghai Medical College, Fudan University, Shanghai, China

Zixiao Yang, MD, PhD Huashan Hospital, Shanghai Medical College, Fudan University, Shanghai, China

Qi Yue, MD, PhD Huashan Hospital, Shanghai Medical College, Fudan University, Shanghai, China

Xin Zhang, MD, PhD Huashan Hospital, Shanghai Medical College, Fudan University, Shanghai, China

Fengping Zhu, MD, PhD Huashan Hospital, Shanghai Medical College, Fudan University, Shanghai, China

Xiang Zou, MD, PhD Huashan Hospital, Shanghai Medical College, Fudan University, Shanghai, China

1 External Carotid Artery-Radial Artery-Middle Cerebral Artery Bypass

Jianping Song, Wei Zhu, and Ying Mao

Abstract

The management of complex internal carotid artery (ICA) aneurysms remains a challenge for vascular neurosurgeons. Because of the giant aneurysm size, fusiform or dissecting morphology, or the presence of many intramural thrombi in some cases, neither endovascular coiling nor microsurgical clipping is optimal, and sacrificing the parent artery may be a better way to treat the aneurysm. Additionally, extracranial–intracranial (EC-IC) vascular bypass is required to reconstruct the blood flow of the middle cerebral artery (MCA) before completely obliterating or trapping the parent artery for the patients with complex aneurysms involving the ICA. The high-flow bypass approach is suitable for treating large or giant ICA aneurysms that cannot be cured by routine endovascular coiling or surgical clipping, especially those originating from the paraclinoid segment, ophthalmic artery (OA), posterior communicating artery (PcomA), or cavernous sinus (CS) segment of the ICA.

Here, we present a case of a giant ICA aneurysms that were treated by an external carotid artery–radial artery-MCA bypass combined with aneurysm trapping.

J. Song · W. Zhu · Y. Mao (✉)
Huashan Hospital, Shanghai Medical College, Fudan University, Shanghai, China
e-mail: maoying@fudan.edu.cn

Keywords

Extracranial–intracranial bypass · Internal carotid artery · Intracranial aneurysm Middle cerebral artery · Radial artery Revascularization

1.1 Introduction

The management of complex internal carotid artery (ICA) aneurysms remains a challenge for vascular neurosurgeons. Because of the giant aneurysm size, fusiform or dissecting morphology, or the presence of many intramural thrombi in some cases, neither endovascular coiling nor microsurgical clipping is optimal, and sacrificing the parent artery may be a better way to treat the aneurysm. Additionally, extracranial–intracranial (EC-IC) vascular bypass is required to reconstruct the blood flow of the middle cerebral artery (MCA) before completely obliterating or trapping the parent artery for the patients with complex aneurysms involving the ICA [1].

This high-flow bypass approach is suitable for treating large or giant ICA aneurysms that cannot be cured by routine endovascular coiling or surgical clipping, especially those originating from the paraclinoid segment, ophthalmic artery (OA), posterior communicating artery (PcomA), or cavernous sinus (CS) segment of the ICA. The com-

Y. Mao et al. (eds.), *Surgical Atlas of Cerebral Revascularization*,
https://doi.org/10.1007/978-981-16-0374-7_1

monly used bypass techniques include high-flow EC-IC (external carotid artery–radial artery–middle cerebral artery, ECA-RA-MCA or external carotid artery–saphenous vein–middle cerebral artery, ECA-SV-MCA) bypass and medium-flow (superficial temporal artery–radial artery–middle cerebral artery, STA-RA-MCA) bypass. Most researchers do not recommend the use of low-flow (STA-MCA) bypass.

We believe that ECA-RA-MCA bypass is the most efficient and safe revascularization technique for giant ICA aneurysms [2].

1.2 Case

A 57-year-old man presented with blurred vision and facial numbness on the left side for 3 months. Physical examination did not reveal hemiparesis, with VOS 0.2 and VOD 0.6. Magnetic resonance imaging (MRI) showed a giant lesion with a prominent flow void sign located in the left CS. Digital subtraction angiography (DSA) revealed a giant left ICA aneurysm (C4 segment) (Fig. 1.1). He could not tolerate a preoperative balloon occlusion test (BOT). Endovascular

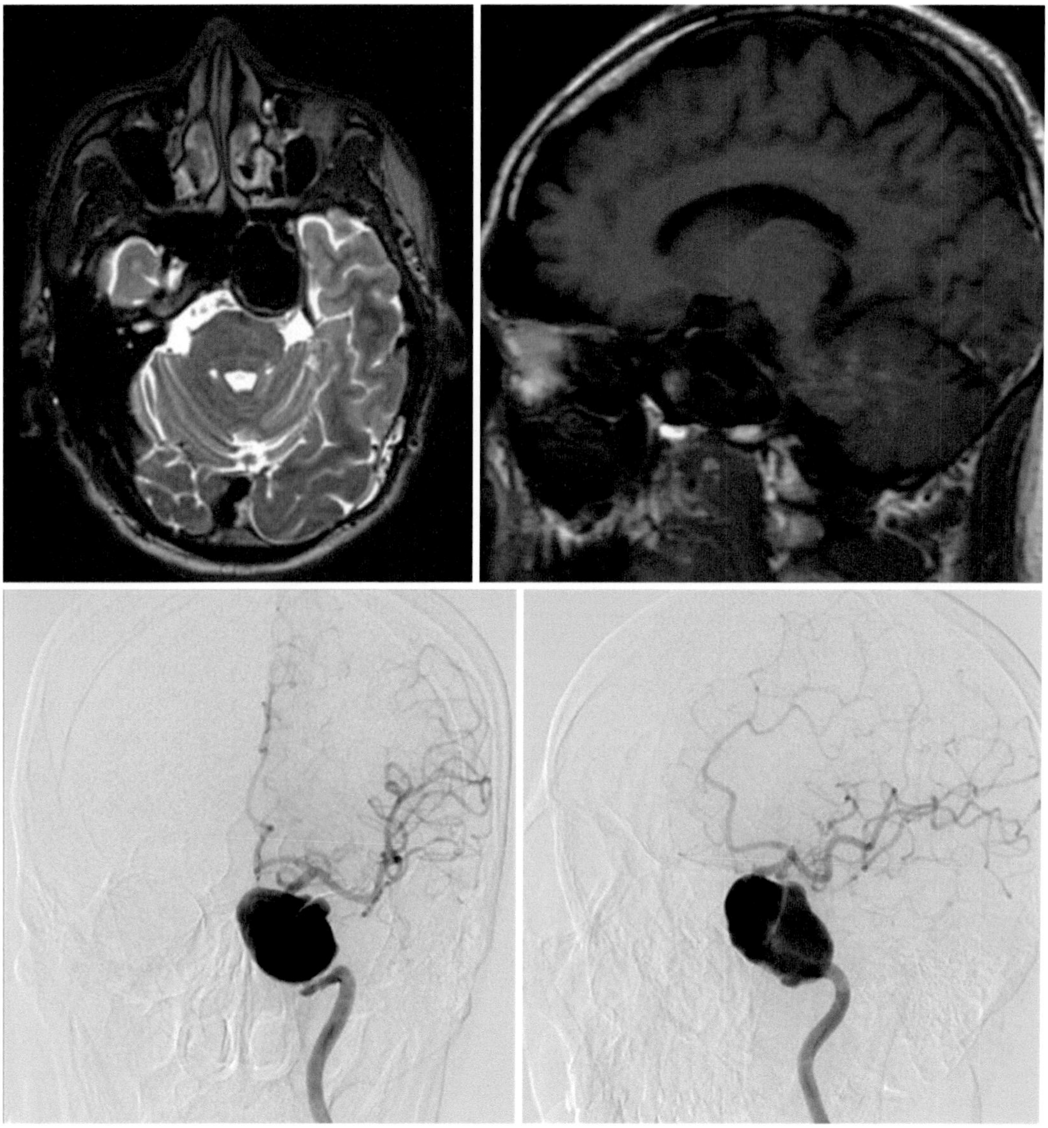

Fig. 1.1 Preoperative imaging: MRI and DSA demonstrated a giant aneurysm in the C4 segment of the left ICA

treatment was difficult for this patient. Therefore, to secure the aneurysm, a left ECA–RA–MCA bypass was planned before occluding the left ICA (Fig. 1.2).

1.3 Details of the Procedure

During the operation, the patient was placed supine with the head turned 45° to the right, and the left shoulder was elevated. The head was elevated by 20° to facilitate venous drainage. His head, neck, and forearm were draped on the left side.

A curvilinear incision was made from the biceps tendon distally toward the wrist crease. The RA was carefully identified and isolated by ligating its branches (Fig. 1.3). After harvesting the RA, the lumen of the RA graft was irrigated with heparinized saline, and the intima edges were trimmed and marked with methylene blue. The "pressure distension" technique was performed for hydrostatic angioplasty (Fig. 1.4), and papaverine was used to treat vasospasm.

After a modified pterional craniotomy, the sylvian fissure was carefully dissected under a microscope, and the M3 branches of the MCA were exposed. One of the M3 branches without perforating vessels was temporarily clipped as the recipient artery. The RA graft was temporarily placed on the recipient M3 vessel to determine the anastomosis site's location and length (marked by methylene blue). A rubber background was placed under the isolated vessel for arteriotomy (Fig. 1.5).

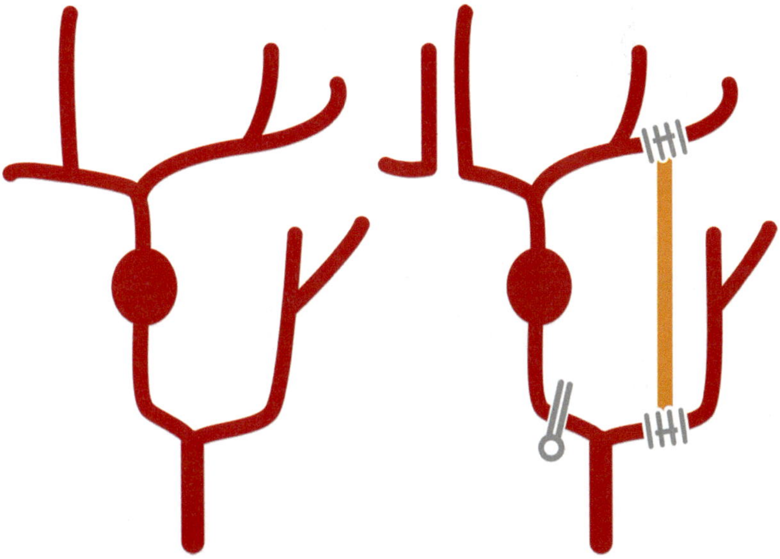

Fig. 1.2 A left ECA-RA-MCA bypass was planned before occluding the left ICA

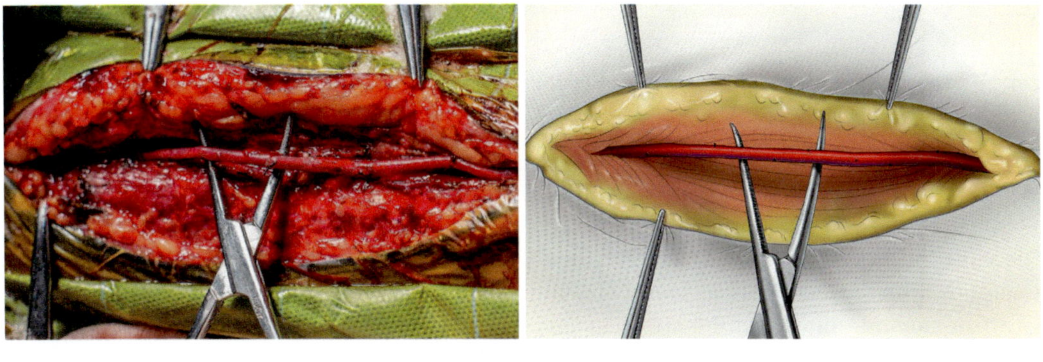

Fig. 1.3 The radial artery (RA) was harvested. The RA was carefully identified and isolated by ligating its branches

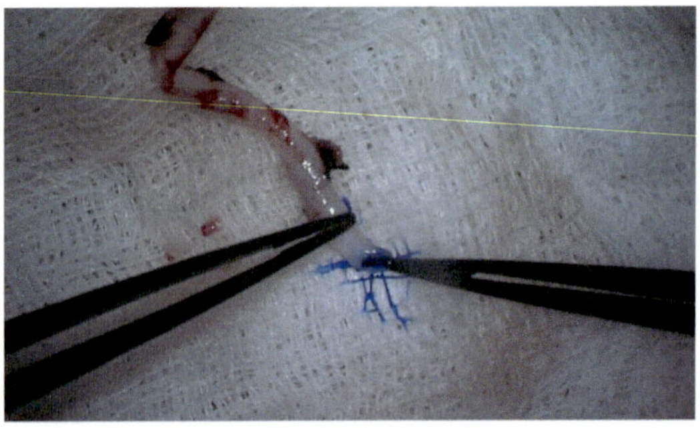
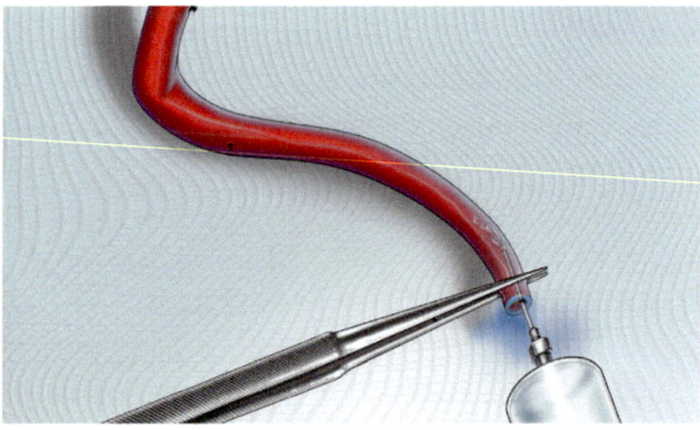

Fig. 1.4 The lumen of the RA graft was irrigated with heparinized saline, and the intima edges were trimmed and marked with methylene blue

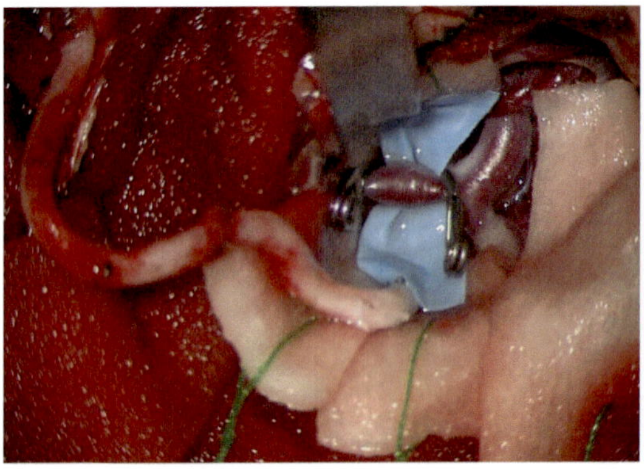
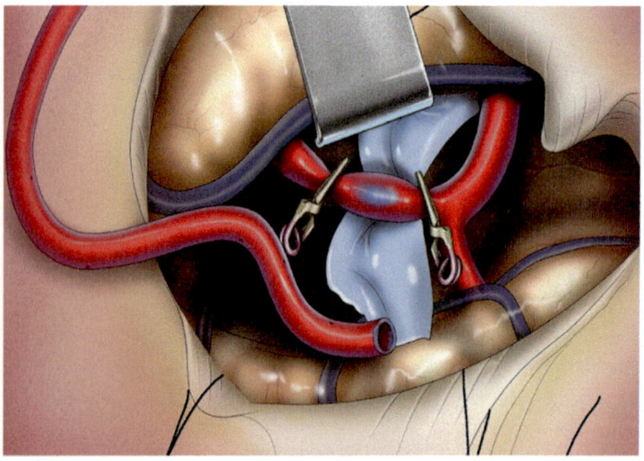

Fig. 1.5 The sylvian fissure was carefully dissected under a microscope, and the M3 branches of the MCA were exposed. One of the M3 branches without perforating vessels was temporarily clipped as the recipient artery

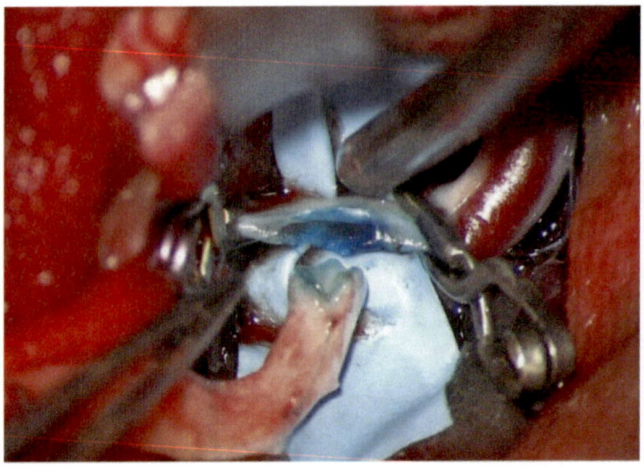
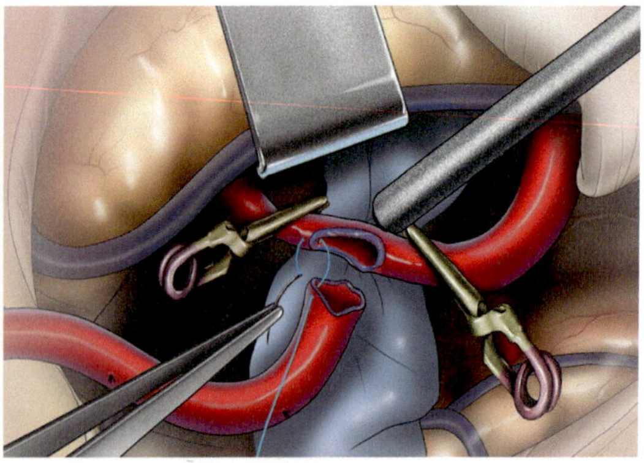

Fig. 1.6 An end-to-side anastomosis strategy was applied for RA graft and recipient M3 suturing. The anastomosis site on the recipient M3 vessel was cut in a fish-mouth fashion, and the anchor suture was placed at the distal corner of the anastomosis

An end-to-side anastomosis was applied for RA graft and recipient M3 suturing. The anastomosis site on the recipient M3 vessel was cut in a fish-mouth fashion, and the artery lumina was irrigated with heparinized saline. The intima edge of the recipient M3 vessel was further marked by methylene blue. The anchor suture was placed at the distal corner of the anastomosis (Fig. 1.6). Then, an opposite anchor suture (180° apart along the vessel circumference) was placed on the anastomosis (Fig. 1.7).

The front wall was sutured interruptedly with 6–8 stitches (Fig. 1.8). The anastomosis was then rotated to expose the back wall for interrupted suturing with 6–8 stitches (Fig. 1.9). The temporary clip was then removed to check for oozing from the anastomotic stoma, and additional stitches were placed to stop the bleeding, if necessary. If no oozing or stenosis of the anastomotic stoma occurred, the RA graft was temporarily clipped, and the recipient M3 vessel was considered patent.

A linear cervical incision was made along the anterior border of the sternocleidomastoid muscle to expose the common carotid artery (CCA)

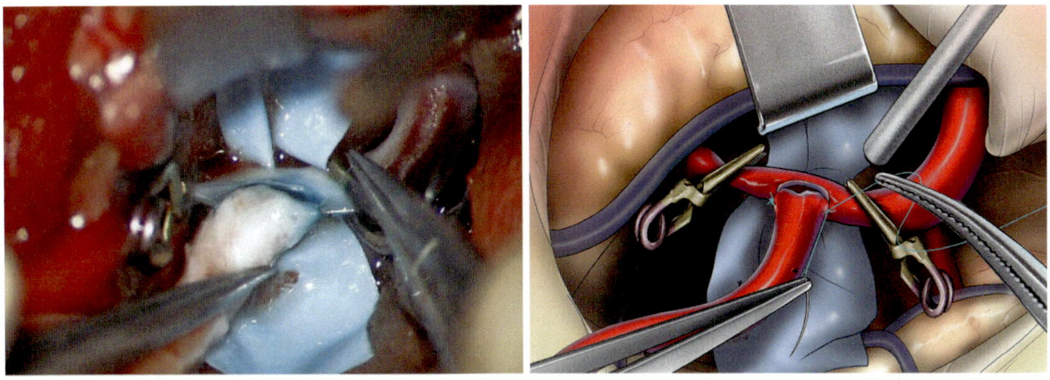

Fig. 1.7 An opposite anchor suture (180° apart along the vessel circumference) was placed on the anastomosis

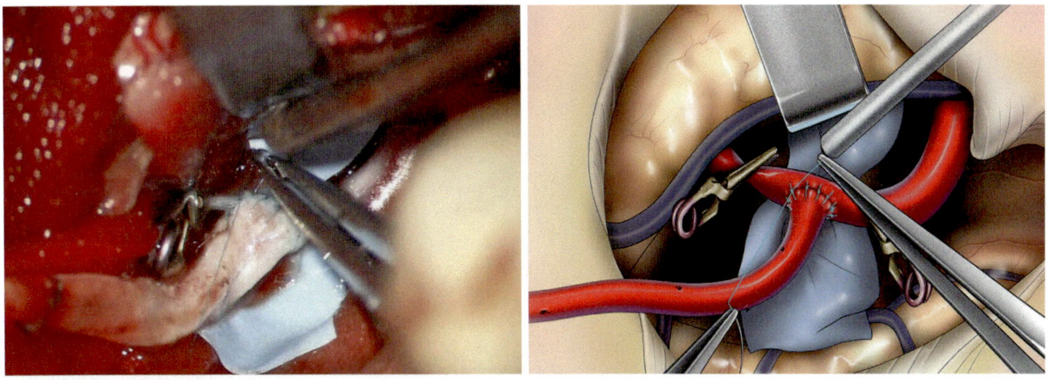

Fig. 1.8 The front wall was sutured interruptedly with 6–8 stitches

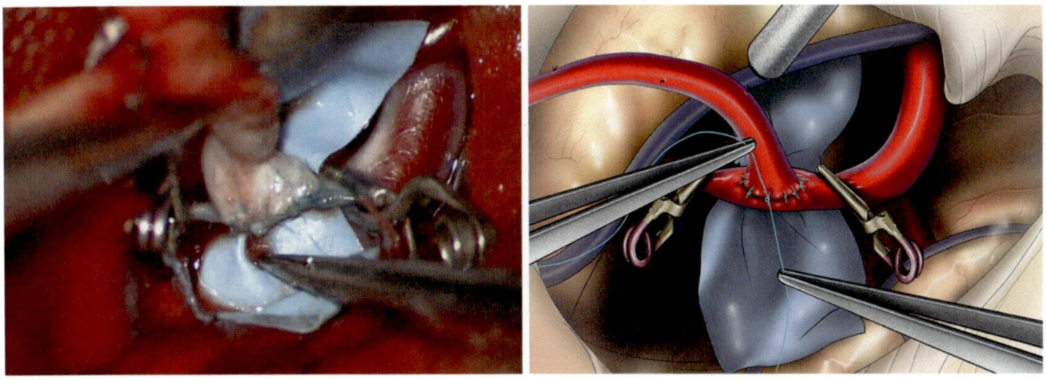

Fig. 1.9 The anastomosis was rotated to expose the back wall, and 6–8 interrupted sutures were placed

and its distal branches (ICA and ECA), respectively. The superior thyroid artery, which originates from the ECA, was also dissected. The RA graft was then led to a cervical incision subcutaneously and cut to the proper length to make it curve naturally without kinking. The ECA and superior thyroid artery were temporarily clamped. A rubber background was placed under the ECA at the anastomosis site, and an arteriotomy was performed. From this point, the lumina of the ECA and superior thyroid artery were flushed with heparinized saline and prepared for anastomosis (Fig. 1.10).

An end-to-side anastomosis was also applied for RA graft and ECA suturing (Fig. 1.11). Two running nonlocking sutures were made for the anastomosis. Stitches were placed 1–2 mm apart in equal intervals. The two-suture technique was used for anastomosis to maintain the vascular tension of the anastomosis stoma and prevent the vessel intima from folding inward. (The first suture needle was passed through both sides but not pulled through, and the stitch was placed by the second suture. Then, the second suture needle was passed through like the first one, which allowed the first suture to be pulled through and tied. This procedure was repeated to place the two sutures.) (Fig. 1.12).

After the RA graft and ECA anastomosis were complete, the temporary clips on the RA graft, ECA, and superior thyroid artery were removed in sequence (Fig. 1.13). Then, the ICA was permanently occluded to trap the aneurysm. In this case, no clip was placed distally to the aneurysm to allow for gradual thrombosis in the distal ICA beyond the occlusion point and prevent unexpected complications due to acute thrombosis.

The Doppler probe was used to confirm the patency of the RA graft and blood flow in the distal recipient vessels (Fig. 1.14).

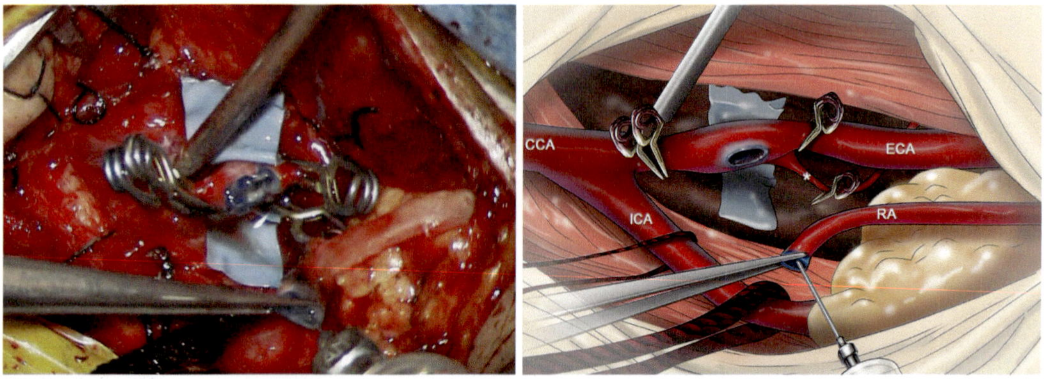

Fig. 1.10 The ECA and superior thyroid artery were temporarily clamped. A rubber background was placed under the ECA at the anastomosis site, and arteriotomy was performed. From this point, the lumina of the ECA and superior thyroid artery (asterisk) were flushed with heparinized saline and prepared for anastomosis

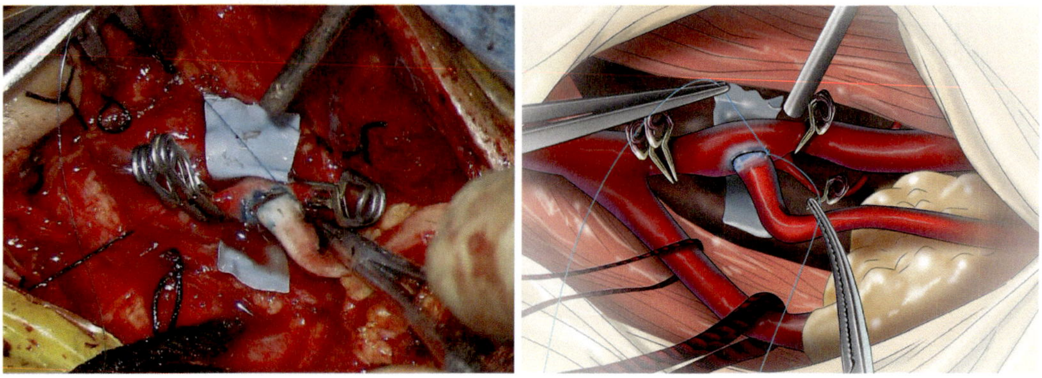

Fig. 1.11 An end-to-side anastomosis was also applied for RA graft and ECA suturing

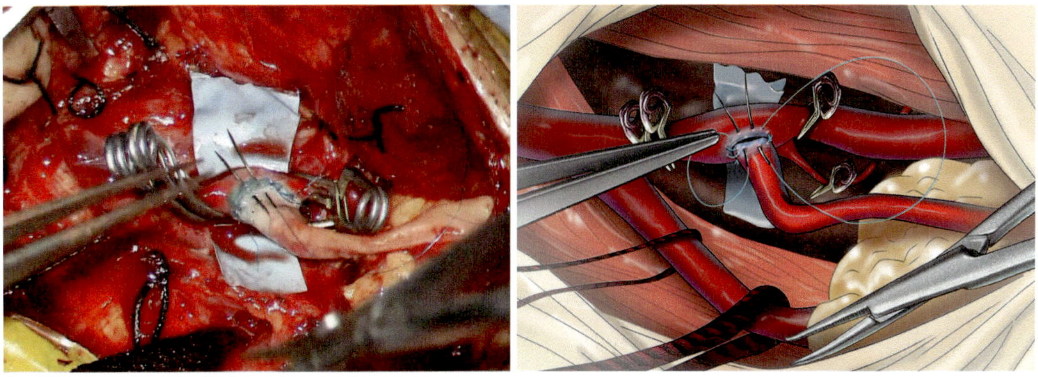

Fig. 1.12 The two-suture technique was used during anastomosis to maintain the vascular tension of the anastomosis stoma and prevent the vessel intima from folding inward

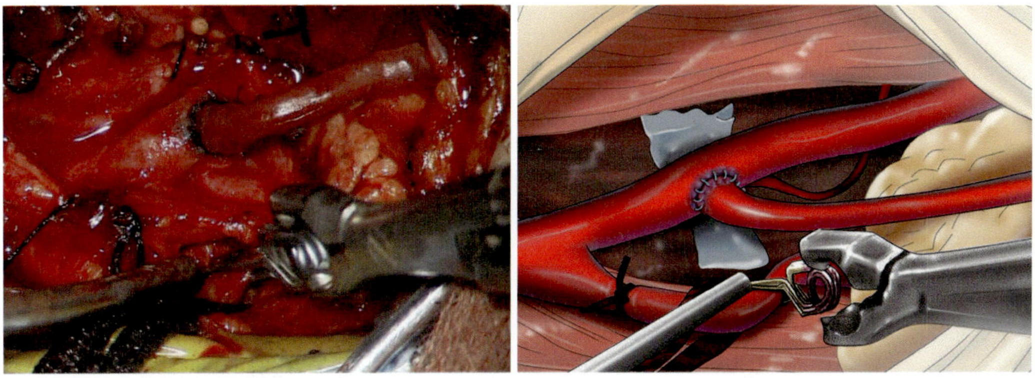

Fig. 1.13 After the RA graft and ECA anastomosis were complete, the temporary clips on the RA graft, ECA, and superior thyroid artery were removed in sequence

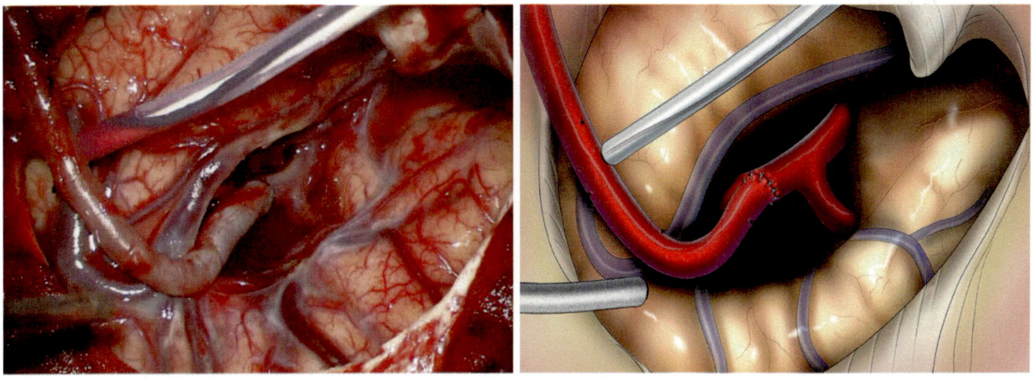

Fig. 1.14 The Doppler probe was used to confirm the patency of the RA graft and the blood flow in the distal recipient vessels

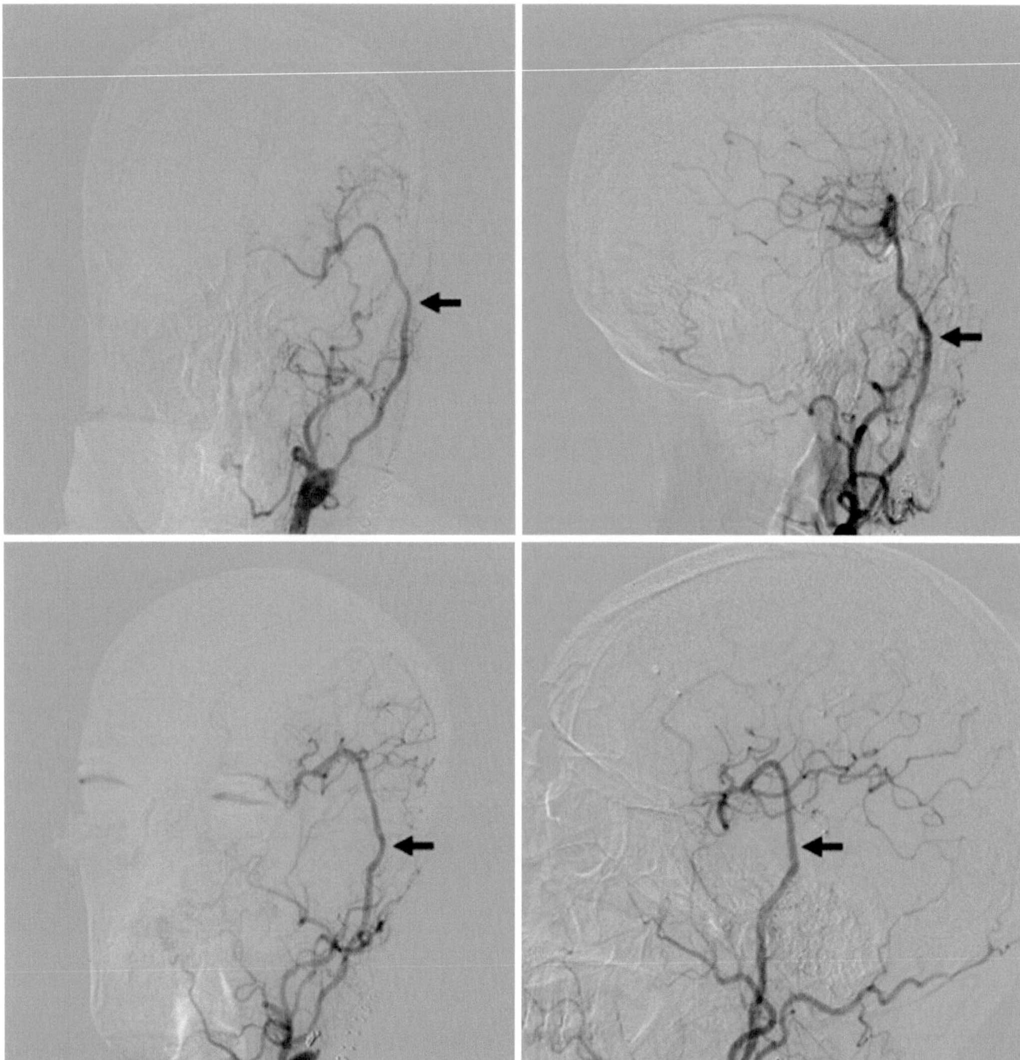

Fig. 1.15 Postoperative DSA showed patency of the RA graft (black arrow) and satisfactory filling of the distal MCA

Postoperative DSA showed patency of the RA graft (black arrow) and satisfactory filling of the distal MCA. (Fig. 1.15).

1.4 Comment

The accurate prediction of the prolonged occlusion tolerance or sacrifice of ICA before operation remains controversial. There is currently no single well-accepted test to accurately predict patients' tolerance to the ICA's permanent occlusion. However, many centers have reported their assessment methods [3–5]. The commonly used method is BOT [3]. Other modalities include enhanced BOT, single-photon emission computed tomography (SPECT), positron emission tomography (PET), computed tomography perfusion imaging (CTP), and xenon-enhanced CT. After BOT, an adequate cerebrovascular reserve is considered indispensable to minimize the ischemic risk after permanent ICA occlusion [3].

The preoperative hemodynamic assessment determines the selection of a bypass approach with an appropriate flow rate. Most vascular neurosurgeons agree that the high-flow EC-IC bypass should be performed before sacrificing the ICA if preoperative BOT is failed [3, 6–10]. The RA or saphenous vein can be used as the graft, and we prefer the RA for revascularization. In high-flow EC-IC bypass, our usual recipient vessels are the MCA M2 or M3 segment. The RA lumen caliber closely approximates our recipient vessels. RA grafts also have several advantages other than saphenous vein grafts: (1) it is easier to harvest; (2) it has a lower incidence of graft failure; and (3) it has superior reliability regarding long-term patency. The main disadvantage of RA is spasm. Therefore, after RA harvesting, we routinely performed the pressure distension technique described by Sekhar et al. [10], to decrease the incidence of graft spasm.

Our proposed bypass selection strategies for complex ICA aneurysms are as follows (Fig. 1.16): Whether patients who pass the 30-min BOT without neurologic deficits should be identified. If they additionally have less than a 0.5-s delay in the ipsilateral hemispheric capillary phase from the contralateral ICA angiography, and no signs of hypoperfusion on the mean transit time (MTT), cerebral blood flow (CBF), and cerebral blood volume (CBV) map during CTP, the patients can accept direct ICA sacrifice without additional EC-IC bypass. If there is no retrograde filling to the aneurysm detected during BOT, we can obliterate ICA by proximal occlusion with detachable balloons or coils, even direct surgical ligation through the neck. However, if the retrograde filling to the aneurysm exists, we have to perform ICA trapping on both sides of the aneurysmal orifice. On the contrary, patients who do not tolerate the 30-min BOT should accept the high-flow EC-IC bypass before ICA sacrifice [2].

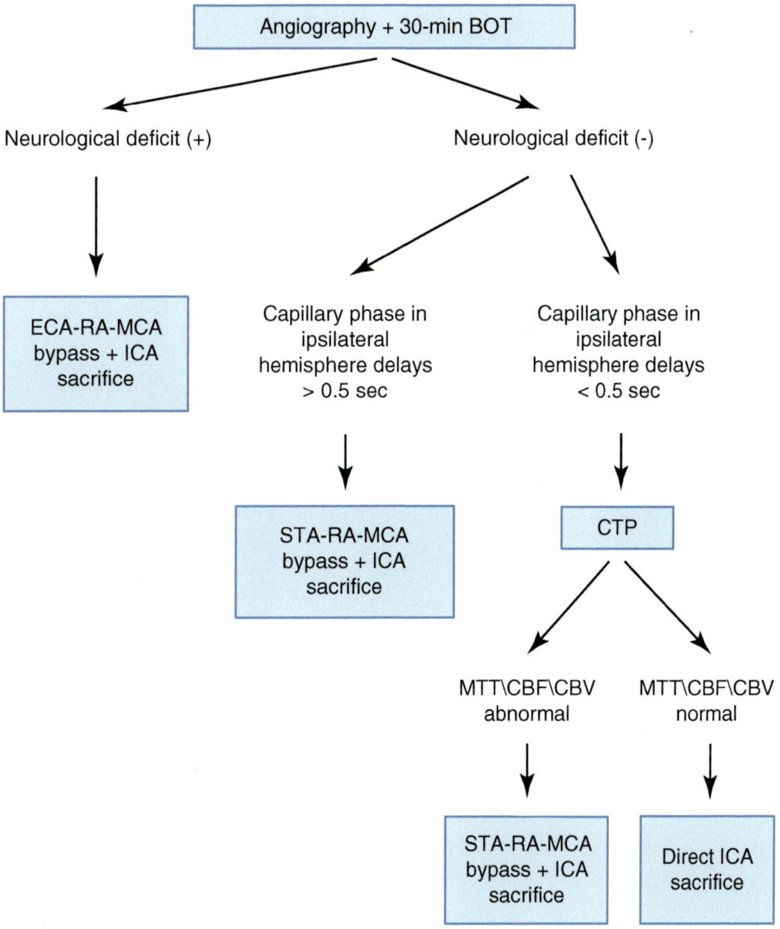

Fig. 1.16 Management algorithm for complex ICA aneurysms (Reproduced from Zhu W, Tian Y, Zhou L, Song D, Xu B, Mao Y. Treatment Strategies for Complex Internal Carotid Artery (ICA) Aneurysms: Direct ICA Sacrifice or Combined with Extracranial-to-Intracranial Bypass. World Neurosurg. 2011; 75(3–4): 476–84.)

References

1. Peerless SJ, Ferguson GG, Drake CG. Extracranial-intracranial (EC/IC) bypass in the treatment of giant intracranial aneurysms. Neurosurg Rev. 1982;5(3):77–81.
2. Zhu W, Tian Y, Zhou L, Song D, Xu B, Mao Y. Treatment strategies for complex internal carotid artery (ICA) aneurysms: direct ICA sacrifice or combined with extracranial-to-intracranial bypass. World Neurosurg. 2011;75(3–4):476–84.
3. Quinones-Hinojosa A, Du R, Lawton MT. Revascularization with saphenous vein bypasses for complex intracranial aneurysms. Skull Base. 2005;15(2):119–32.
4. Wanebo JE, Zabramski JM, Spetzler RF. Superficial temporal artery-to-middle cerebral artery bypass grafting for cerebral revascularization. Neurosurgery. 2004;55(2):395–8. 398-99
5. Sen C, Sekhar LN. Direct vein graft reconstruction of the cavernous, petrous, and upper cervical internal carotid artery: lessons learned from 30 cases. Neurosurgery. 1992;30(5):732–42. 742–43
6. Kai Y, Hamada J, Morioka M, Yano S, Mizuno T, Kuroda J, Todaka T, Takeshima H, Kuratsu J. Treatment strategy for giant aneurysms in the cavernous portion of the internal carotid artery. Surg Neurol. 2007;67(2):148–55. 155
7. Mohit AA, Sekhar LN, Natarajan SK, Britz GW, Ghodke B. High-flow bypass grafts in the management of complex intracranial aneurysms. Neurosurgery. 2007;60(2 Suppl 1):S105–22. S122–23
8. Lawton MT, Quinones-Hinojosa A, Chang EF, Yu T. Thrombotic intracranial aneurysms: classification scheme and management strategies in 68 patients. Neurosurgery. 2005;56(3):441–54. 441–54
9. Ponce FA, Albuquerque FC, McDougall CG, Han PP, Zabramski JM, Spetzler RF. Combined endovascular and microsurgical management of giant and complex unruptured aneurysms. Neurosurg Focus. 2004;17(5):E11.
10. Sekhar LN, Duff JM, Kalavakonda C, Olding M. Cerebral revascularization using radial artery grafts for the treatment of complex intracranial aneurysms: techniques and outcomes for 17 patients. Neurosurgery. 2001;49(3):646–58. 658–59

Superficial Temporal Artery-Radial Artery-Middle Cerebral Artery Bypass

2

Peiliang Li, Liang Chen, Wei Zhu, and Ying Mao

Abstract

Hemodynamic differences are significant in giant aneurysms located in different middle cerebral artery (MCA) segments, and the treatment strategy should be adjusted accordingly. M1 aneurysms that involve important perforating branches such as the lenticulostriate arteries cannot be directly clipped. A moderate- (superficial temporal artery-radial artery-MCA, STA-RA-MCA) or high-flow (external carotid artery-radial artery-MCA, ECA-RA-MCA) extracranial-intracranial (EC-IC) bypass can be combined with aneurysm trapping as an efficient treatment strategy.

Here, we present a case of a giant MCA M1 dissecting aneurysm that was treated by STA-RA-MCA bypass combined with aneurysm trapping.

Keywords

Extracranial-intracranial bypass · Intracranial aneurysm · Middle cerebral artery · Radial artery · Superficial temporal artery Revascularization

P. Li · L. Chen · W. Zhu · Y. Mao (✉)
Huashan Hospital, Shanghai Medical College, Fudan University, Shanghai, China
e-mail: maoying@fudan.edu.cn

2.1 Introduction

Hemodynamic differences are significant in giant aneurysms located in different middle cerebral artery (MCA) segments, and the treatment strategy should be adjusted accordingly. M1 aneurysms that involve important perforating branches such as the lenticulostriate arteries cannot be directly clipped. A moderate- (superficial temporal artery-radial artery-MCA, STA-RA-MCA) or high-flow (external carotid artery-radial artery-MCA, ECA-RA-MCA) extracranial-intracranial (EC-IC) bypass can be combined with aneurysm trapping as an efficient treatment strategy. Due to early thrombosis development in the giant aneurysm and the gradual decrease in intra-aneurysm blood flow, complete thrombosis of the aneurysm can be achieved in most cases [1, 2].

Intraoperative electrophysiological monitoring, including motor evoked potentials (MEPs) and somatosensory evoked potentials (SEPs), plays a vital role in assessing tolerance to vascular occlusion and the timely identification of motor dysfunction due to various causes. Such monitoring is an essential safeguard for MCA aneurysm procedures [3].

Here, we present a case of a giant MCA M1 dissecting aneurysm that was treated by STA-RA-MCA bypass combined with aneurysm trapping.

Y. Mao et al. (eds.), *Surgical Atlas of Cerebral Revascularization*,
https://doi.org/10.1007/978-981-16-0374-7_2

2.2 Case

A 37-year-old woman presented with repeated dizziness for half a year. Physical examination did not reveal any neurological deficits. Magnetic resonance imaging (MRI) and digital subtraction angiography (DSA) demonstrated a left giant MCA (M1) dissecting aneurysm (Fig. 2.1). Endovascular treatment was not suitable for this patient. Therefore, to secure the aneurysm, left STA-RA-MCA bypass combined with proximal occlusion was planned (Fig. 2.2). The reflux from the distal MCA through a bypass graft ensured sufficient blood flow in the lenticulostriate arteries.

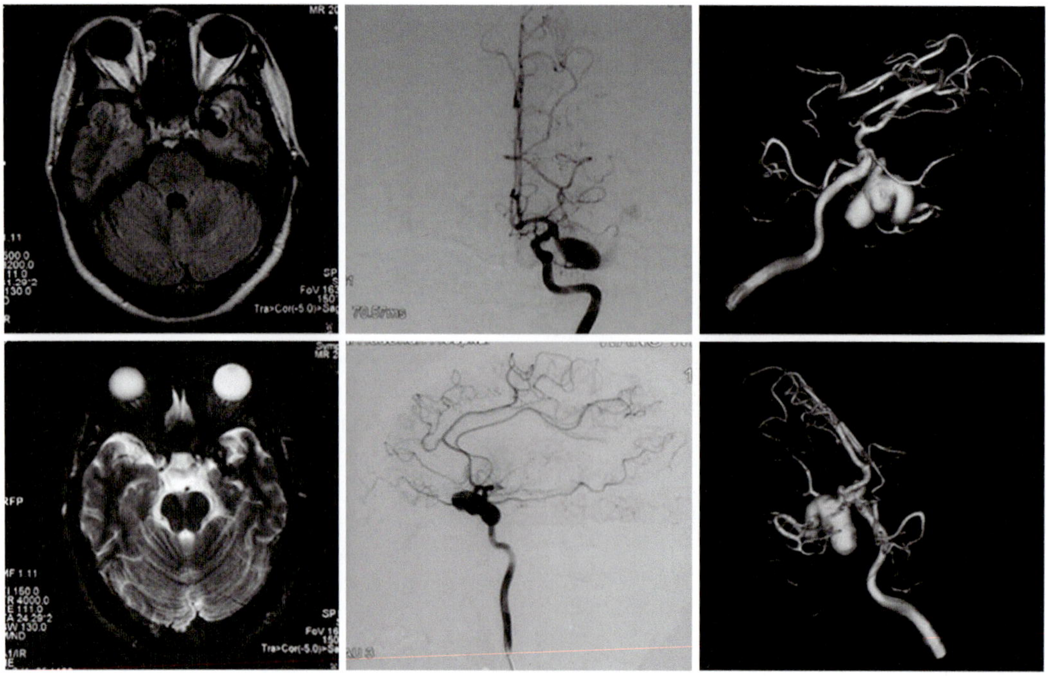

Fig. 2.1 Preoperative imaging: MRI and DSA demonstrated a left giant MCA (M1) dissecting aneurysm

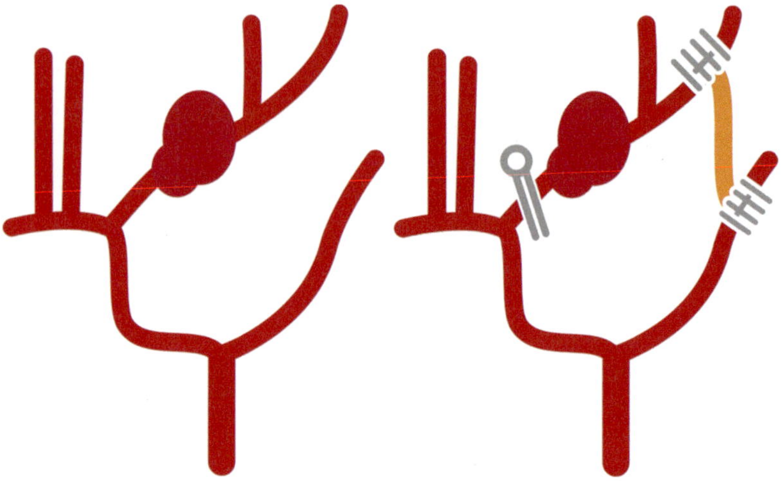

Fig. 2.2 Surgical plan: Left STA-RA-MCA bypass combined with proximal occlusion

2.3 Details of the Procedure

During the operation, the patient was placed supine with the head turned 45° to the right, and the left shoulder elevated. The head was elevated by 20° to facilitate venous drainage. Her head, neck, and forearm were draped on the left side.

The RA graft was harvested and prepared, as described in Chap. 1. A modified pterional craniotomy was performed, and the sylvian fissure was dissected to achieve exposure of the aneurysm and M1 and M2 segments of the MCA (Fig. 2.3). Ideally, the recipient M2 segment should have no branched or perforating vessels (Fig. 2.4).

The recipient M2 segment was temporarily occluded, and a fish-mouth arteriotomy was performed (Fig. 2.5). The graft vessel's lumen was flushed with heparinized saline, and the intima edges were marked with methylene blue. The proximal end of the RA graft was anastomosed to the recipient M2 vessel. A heel stitch was placed at one anchor of the anastomosis, and knots were tied on the outside of the lumen. A toe stitch was placed on the opposite anchor (Fig. 2.6). Interrupted suturing was achieved first on one wall of the anastomosis, ideally with 6–8 stitches (Fig. 2.7). The suture intervals must be consistent. The RA graft was then carefully rotated, and interrupted suturing of the opposite edge of the anastomosis was achieved using the two-suture method (Fig. 2.8). The temporary clips were then removed to check for oozing or stenosis at the site of the anastomosis. Additional stitches might be necessary to achieve a watertight anastomosis.

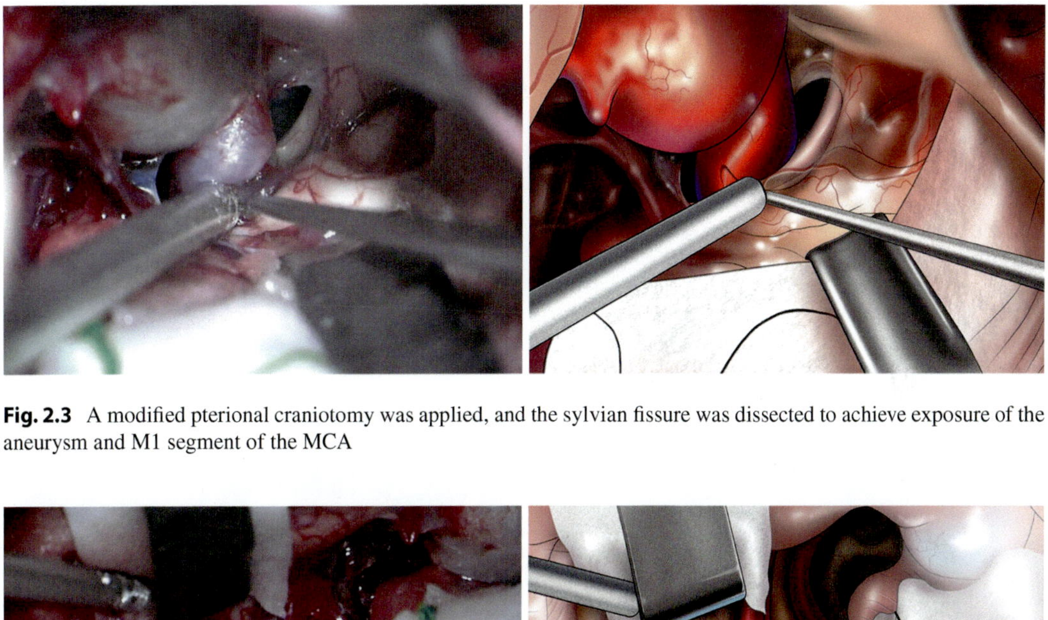

Fig. 2.3 A modified pterional craniotomy was applied, and the sylvian fissure was dissected to achieve exposure of the aneurysm and M1 segment of the MCA

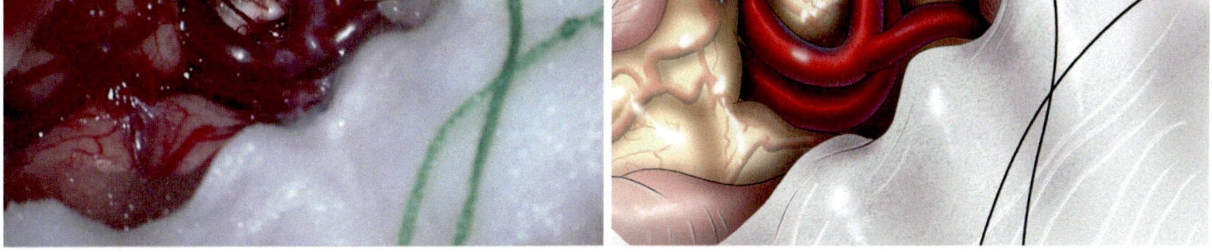

Fig. 2.4 The sylvian fissure was dissected under a microscope, and the M2 branches of the MCA were exposed. Ideally, the recipient M2 segment should have no branched or perforating vessels

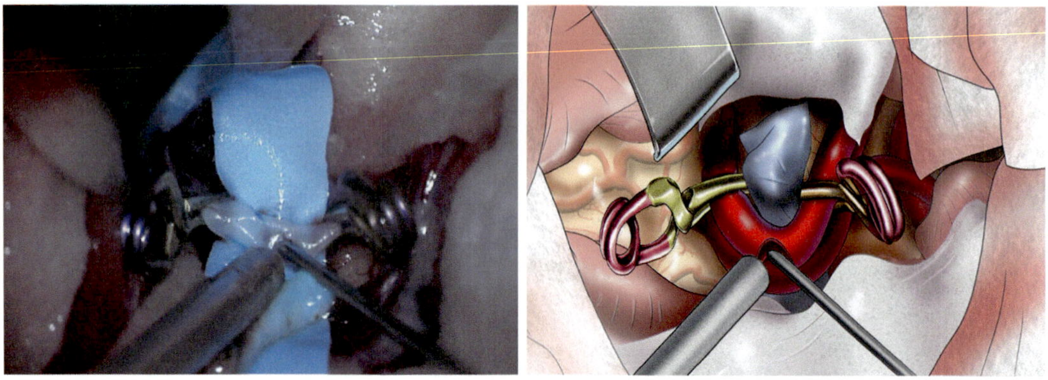

Fig. 2.5 The recipient M2 segment was temporarily occluded, and a fish-mouth arteriotomy was performed

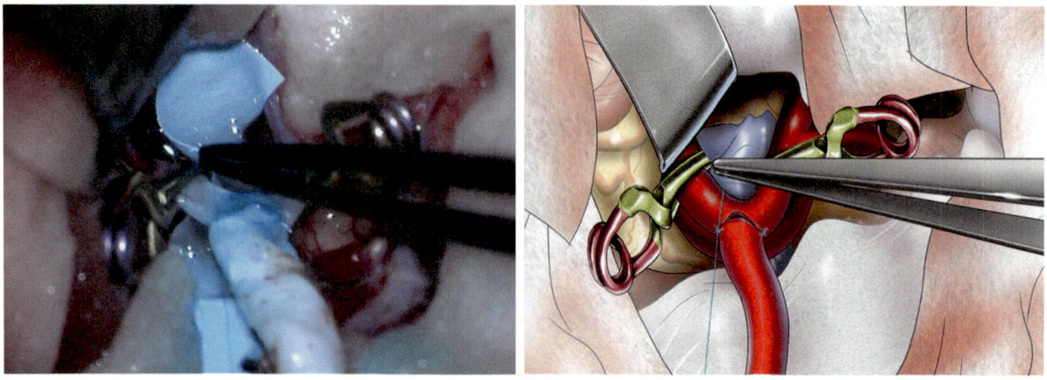

Fig. 2.6 The proximal end of the RA graft was anastomosed to the recipient M2 vessel. A heel stitch was placed at one anchor of the anastomosis, and knots were tied on the outside of the lumen. A toe stitch was placed on the opposite anchor

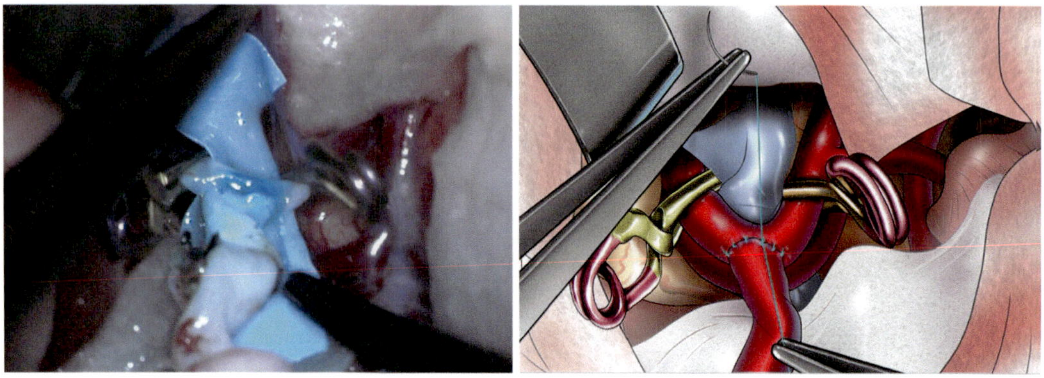

Fig. 2.7 Interrupted suturing was performed first on one wall of the anastomosis, ideally with 6–8 stitches

The graft vessel was then temporarily occluded, and the recipient M2 branch was kept patent (Fig. 2.9).

A sufficient length of the STA trunk was dissected free. The distal portion of the artery was occluded temporarily (Fig. 2.10). Following dis-

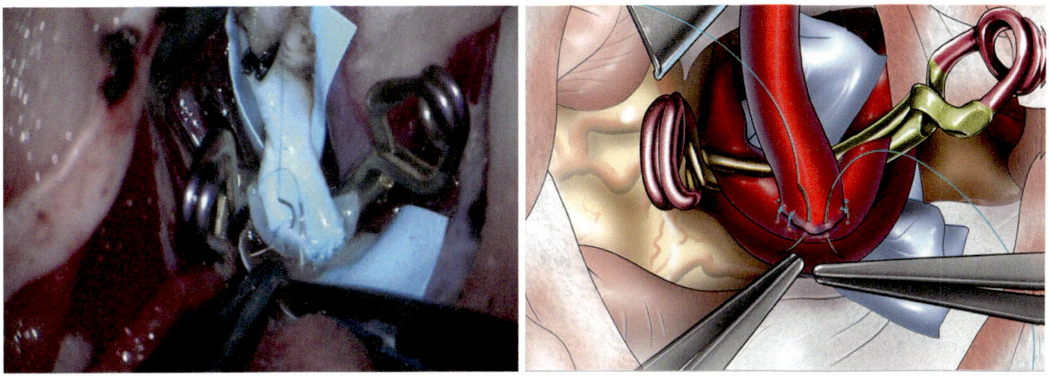

Fig. 2.8 The RA graft was then carefully rotated, and interrupted suturing of the opposite edge of the anastomosis was achieved using the two-suture method

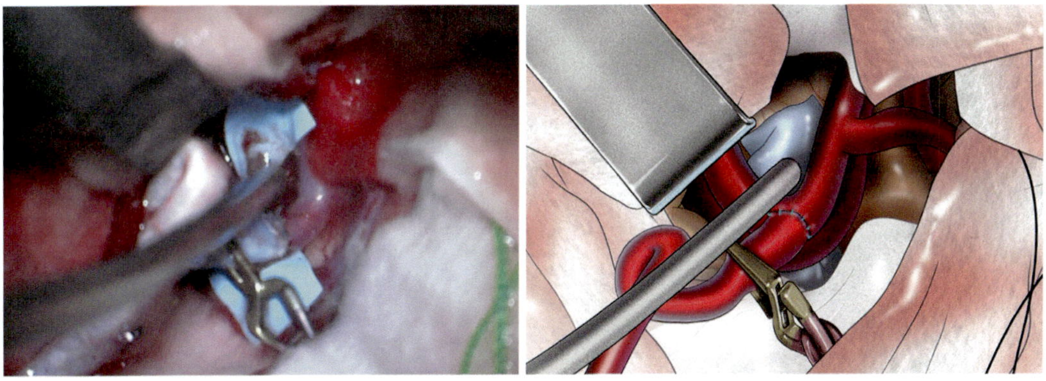

Fig. 2.9 The temporary clips were then removed to check for oozing or stenosis at the site of the anastomosis. The graft vessel was then temporarily occluded, and the recipient M2 branch was kept patent

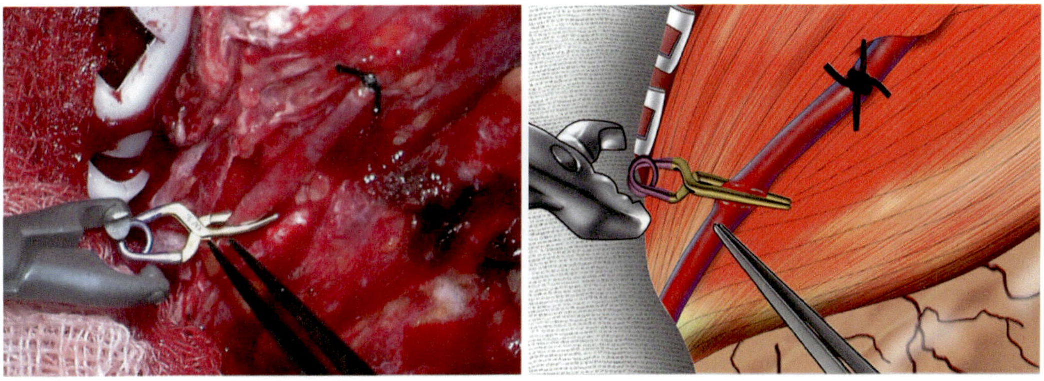

Fig. 2.10 A sufficient length of the STA trunk was dissected free. The distal portion of the artery was occluded temporarily

section and isolation, the STA was then pulled through the temporalis (Fig. 2.11). An end-to-end anastomosis was performed for the STA (donor) and RA (graft) vessels. Two opposite sutures were placed first. The back wall of the anastomosis was sutured interruptedly with 3–4 sutures

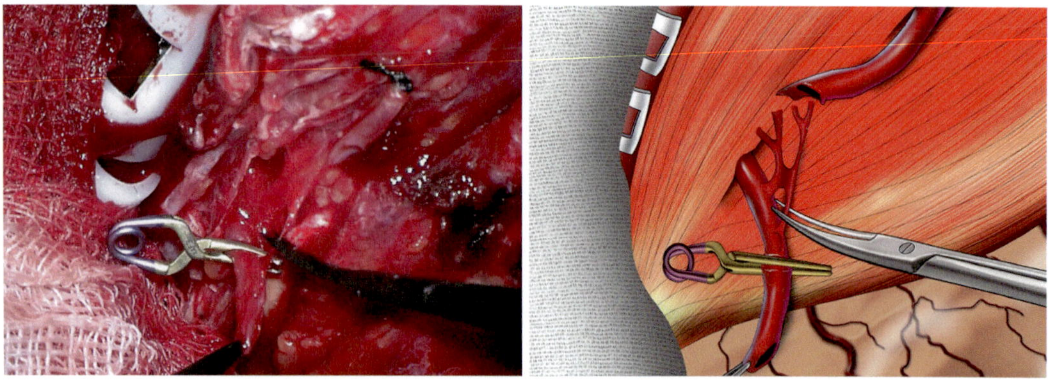

Fig. 2.11 Following dissection and isolation, the STA was then pulled through the temporalis

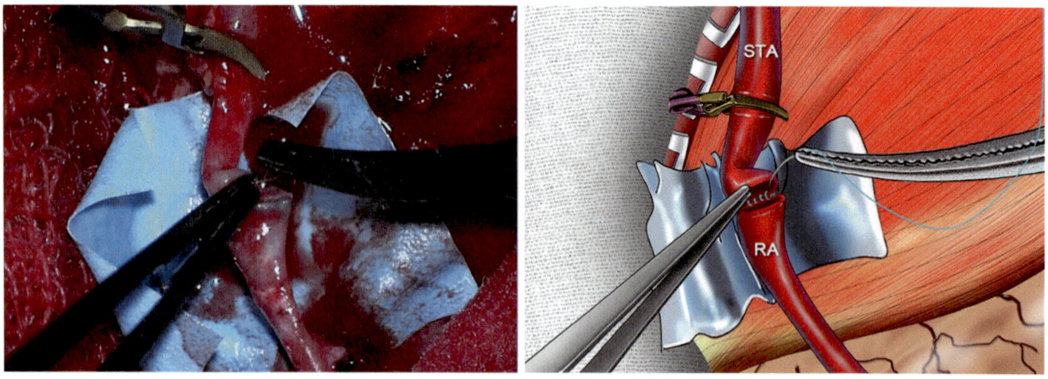

Fig. 2.12 An end-to-end anastomosis was performed for the STA (donor) and RA (graft) vessels. Two opposite sutures were placed first. The back wall of the anastomosis was sutured interruptedly with 3–4 sutures

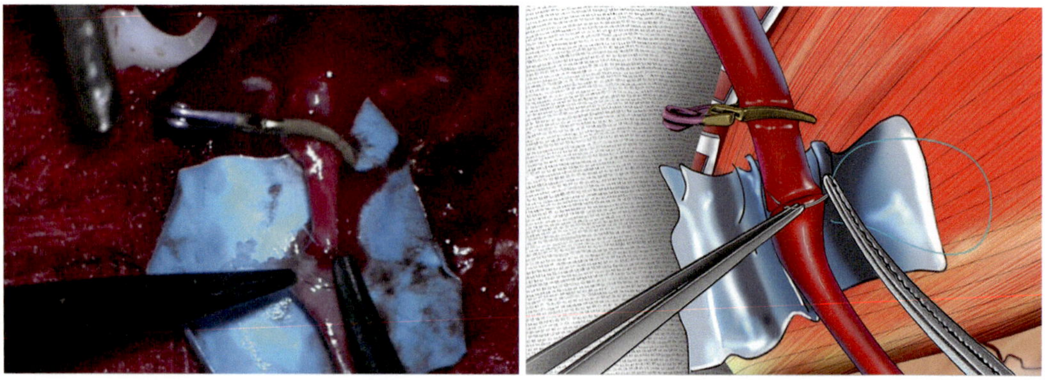

Fig. 2.13 After sutures were placed in the back wall, the vessels were gently rotated to suture the front wall in a similar interrupted fashion with 3–4 sutures

(Fig. 2.12). After sutures were places in the back wall, the vessels were gently rotated to suture the front wall in a similar interrupted fashion with 3–4 sutures (Fig. 2.13).

After STA-RA-MCA bypass was complete, the M1 was clipped permanently proximal to the aneurysm (Fig. 2.14). The temporary clips on the RA graft were removed. A Doppler ultrasound

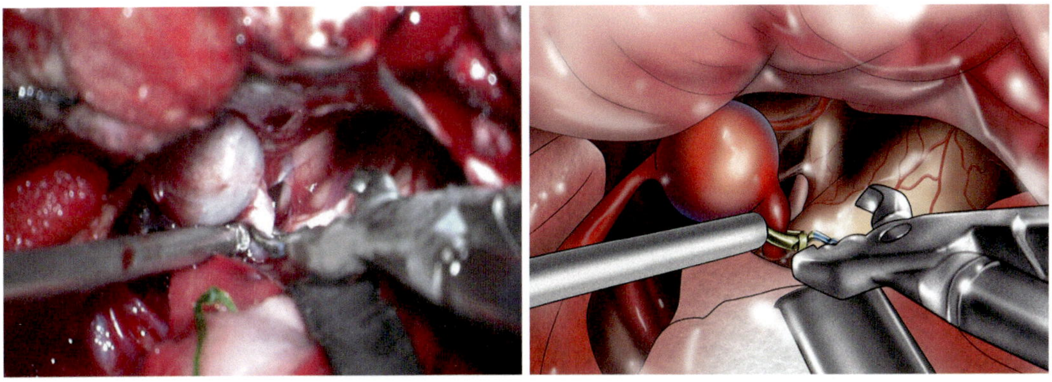

Fig. 2.14 The M1 was clipped permanently proximal to the aneurysm

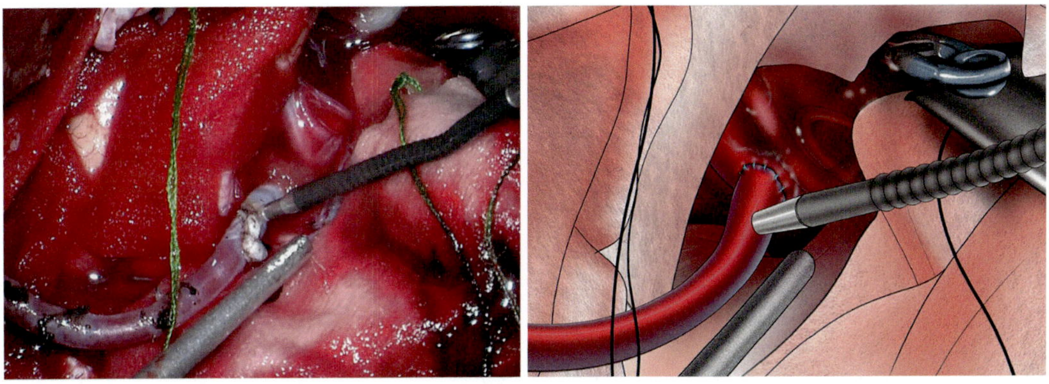

Fig. 2.15 The temporary clips on the RA graft were removed. A Doppler ultrasound probe was utilized to ensure patency of the graft and recipient vessels

probe was utilized to ensure patency of the graft and recipient vessels (Fig. 2.15).

Postoperative DSA showed patency of the RA graft and satisfactory filling of the distal MCA (Fig. 2.16).

2.4 Comment

Complex MCA aneurysms usually cannot be treated with direct clipping or simple coiling due to their large or giant, fusiform, dissecting, broad-necked, or serpentine morphology. The common clinical presentation of complex MCA includes hemorrhage, epilepsy, mass effects, or even cerebral ischemia. These aneurysms may also be incidentally diagnosed without any symptoms. Once ruptured, the patient had an extremely high mortality rate of 65–85% within 2 years [4, 5]. The survivors often suffered from severe neurological sequelae.

The diversity of complex MCA aneurysm morphologies, locations, and hemodynamics required the surgeons to tailor their treatment strategy in each case. However, the aneurysm trapping/resection after the revascularization is a common idea for curing these lesions. We tailored our revascularization strategy based on our 3-type classification of complex MCA aneurysms [2] (Fig. 2.17). The type A aneurysm originates from the M1 segment, type B from the M2 segment/MCA bifurcation, and type C from the M3/distal segments.

The lenticulostriate perforators are often encountered in the base or dome in type A aneurysm, which is a significant challenge for surgical

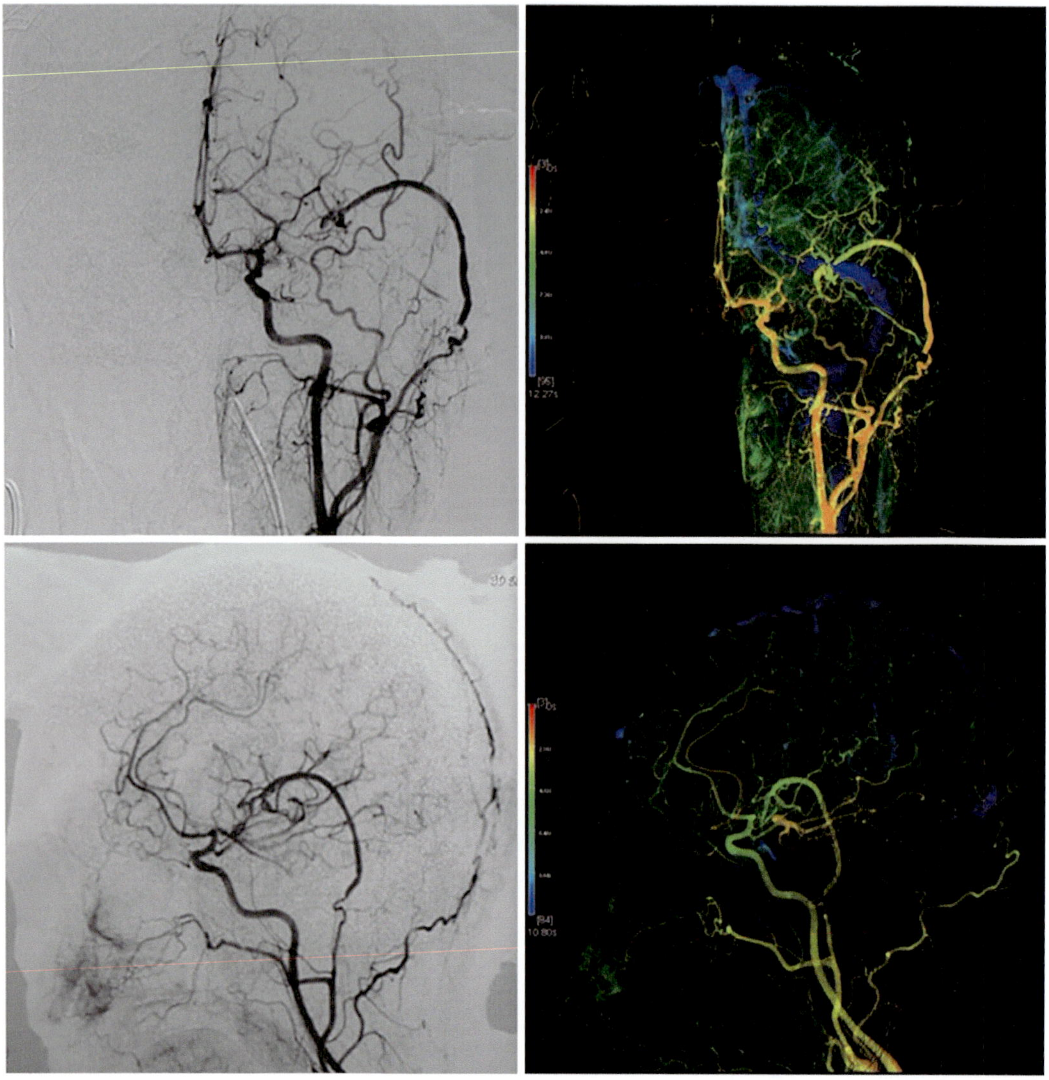

Fig. 2.16 Postoperative DSA showed patency of the RA graft and satisfactory filling of the distal MCA

treatment. If the perforators are not involved in the aneurysm's neck, direct clipping is applicable with perforator preservation. However, if the perforators originated from the aneurysmal neck or dome, direct clipping/trapping may cause inevitable damage to them, even after distal revascularization. Therefore, we advocated for STA-RA-MCA bypass in treating type A aneurysm, followed by ICA sacrifice (only proximal trapping) without complete aneurysm trapping. This strategy may not achieve immediate aneurysm obliteration, but the postsurgical hemodynamic change due to significantly reduced blood filling into the aneurysm can initiate aneurysm thrombosis and lead to a lower rupture risk rupture. Therefore, this strategy is usually considered as a protective procedure. Although thrombosis may occlude the lenticulostriate perforators, the occlusion is usually a delayed course, generating an "ischemic preconditioning" environment for the involved neurons. The potential collateral circulation was also promoted. Alaraj et al. reported that the STA trunk's flow capacity was high (54–100 ml/min), and the RA graft's flow ranged from 50 to 70 ml/min [6], supporting the circulation in the MCA supplying

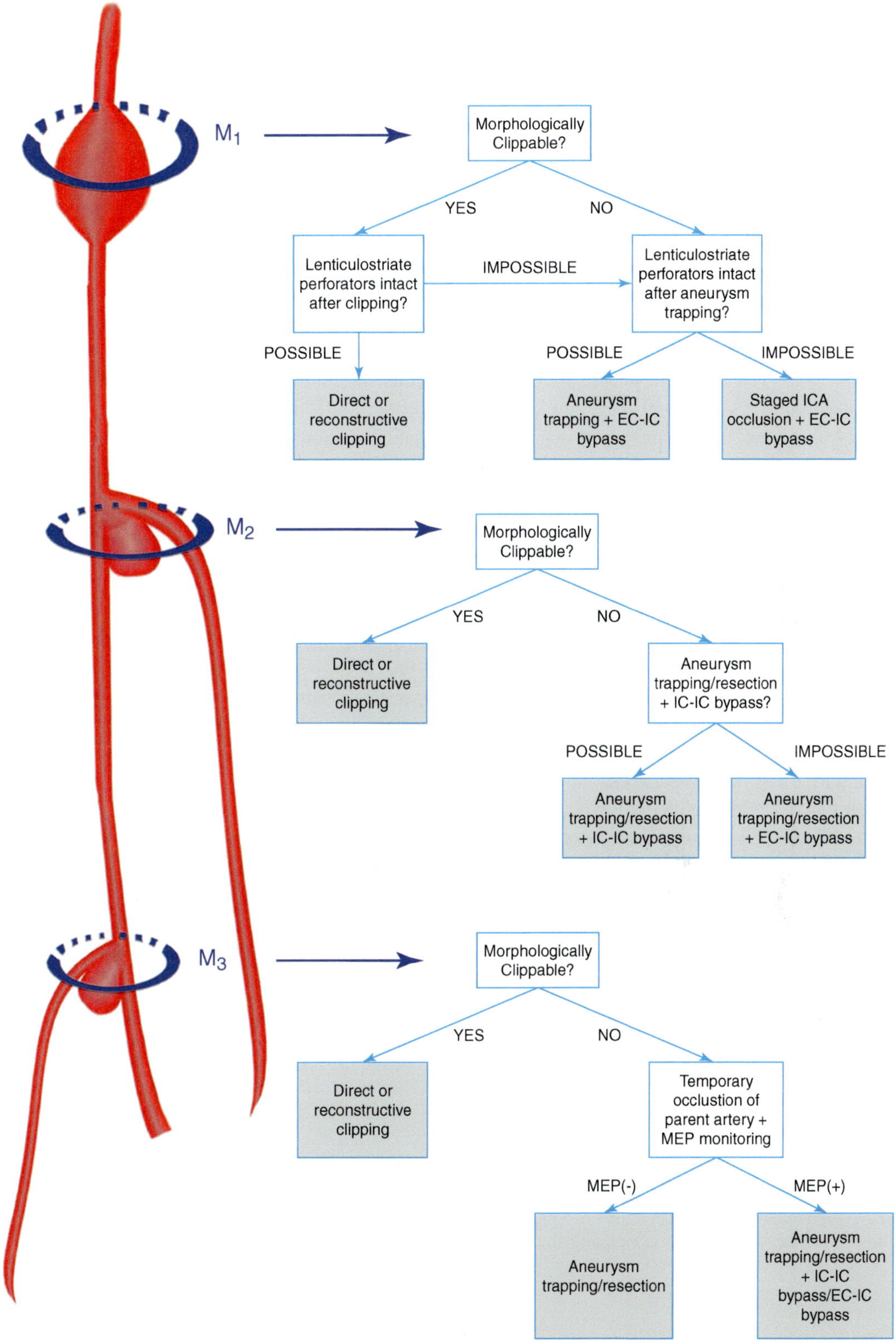

Fig. 2.17 The algorithm of our surgical strategies for treating complex MCA aneurysms (Reproduced from Zhu W, Liu P, Tian Y, Gu Y, Xu B, Chen L, Zhou L, Mao Y. Complex middle cerebral artery aneurysms: a new classification based on the angioarchitecture and surgical strategies. Acta Neurochir. 2013; 155(8): 1481–91.)

area sufficiently. Therefore, this middle-flow bypass (STA-RA-MCA) approach is suitable for treating large or giant proximal MCA aneurysms that are not suitable for endovascular coiling or surgical clipping, especially giant serpentine aneurysms, dissecting aneurysms, or M1 aneurysms.

For type B aneurysm cases, if trapping will be conducted to obliterate the aneurysm, a revascularization strategy should be performed. The morphology of complex aneurysms at the M1–M2 bifurcation is usually fusiform without a clear neck. In that case, one of the M2 branches may be preserved using the reconstructive clipping technique. For a giant aneurysm with significant thrombus inside, aneurysm opening and thrombus removal using an ultrasonic aspirator may be required for mass effect decompression and reconstructive clipping. If oozing occurs during thrombus removal, it can be controlled using a cottonoid patty compression technique or proximal temporary occlusion in the parent artery. During aneurysm dissection, the surgeons should do their best to preserve the adjacent arterial branches, especially the lenticulostriate perforators. However, if clipping is not applicable, aneurysm trapping with one of the M2 branches sacrificing will be considered. Some studies report that one of the M2 branches occlusion may not lead to postoperative cerebral ischemia without bypass in selected cases, but the precise predictor is lacking. Therefore, we suggest revascularization should be performed in all type B aneurysms if one of the M2 will be sacrificed. The revascularization strategy includes EC-IC bypass (STA-RA-M3 bypass, STA-M3 bypass) or intracranial-intracranial bypass (side-to-side M3–M3 bypass, in situ M2–M2 anastomosis) [7, 8]. At last, the aneurysm can be trapped or even resected for decompression.

The aneurysm obliteration using simple parent artery sacrifice is usually tolerable in most type C aneurysms. However, if the aneurysms are located at the central arteries or angular arteries supplying the eloquent cortex, these arteries' occlusion may result in postoperative neurological sequelae. A low-flow bypass, like STA-M3 bypass or in situ M3–M3 anastomosis, is mandatory before aneurysm trapping or resection. The necessity of revascularization can also be estimated based on routine intraoperative MEPs and SEPs monitoring techniques for type C aneurysms [6]. During the 20-min parent artery temporary occlusion, if significant decrement of MEPs and SEPs signal occurs, the revascularization is highly indicated; otherwise, we may directly occlude the parent artery. However, surgeons should be aware that this technique is not appropriate if the parent artery supplying eloquent language or optical area, which cannot be monitored by MEPs or SEPs.

References

1. Zhu W, Mao Y. Treatment of unruptured middle cerebral artery aneurysms: the risk factors and surgical safety. World Neurosurg. 2015;84(3):618–9.
2. Zhu W, Liu P, Tian Y, Gu Y, Xu B, Chen L, Zhou L, Mao Y. Complex middle cerebral artery aneurysms: a new classification based on the angioarchitecture and surgical strategies. Acta Neurochir. 2013;155(8):1481–91.
3. Yue Q, Zhu W, Gu Y, Xu B, Lang L, Song J, Cai J, Xu G, Chen L, Mao Y. Motor evoked potential monitoring during surgery of middle cerebral artery aneurysms: a cohort study. World Neurosurg. 2014;82(6):1091–9.
4. Choi IS, David C. Giant intracranial aneurysms: development, clinical presentation and treatment. Eur J Radiol. 2003;46(3):178–94.
5. Drake CG, Peerless SJ. Giant fusiform intracranial aneurysms: review of 120 patients treated surgically from 1965 to 1992. J Neurosurg. 1997;87(2):141–62.
6. Alaraj A, Ashley WJ, Charbel FT, Amin-Hanjani S. The superficial temporal artery trunk as a donor vessel in cerebral revascularization: benefits and pitfalls. Neurosurg Focus. 2008;24(2):E7.
7. Seo BR, Kim TS, Joo SP, Lee JM, Jang JW, Lee JK, Kim JH, Kim SH. Surgical strategies using cerebral revascularization in complex middle cerebral artery aneurysms. Clin Neurol Neurosurg. 2009;111(8):670–5.
8. Tayebi MA, Huang W, Benet A, Kola O, Lawton MT. Bypass surgery for complex middle cerebral artery aneurysms: an algorithmic approach to revascularization. J Neurosurg. 2017;127(3):463–79.

Superficial Temporal Artery-Middle Cerebral Artery Bypass

3

Yujun Liao, Wei Ni, Liang Chen, and Bin Xu

Abstract

Superficial temporal artery-middle cerebral artery (STA-MCA) bypass, developed and popularized by Yasargil and Donaghy in the late 1960s, remains the most straightforward and versatile extracranial-intracranial (EC-IC) bypass method today, with applications in treating Moyamoya disease, cerebral aneurysms, and intracranial atherosclerosis.

Keywords

Extracranial-intracranial bypass · Intracranial aneurysm · Middle cerebral artery Moyamoya disease · Superficial temporal artery · Revascularization

3.1 Introduction

Superficial temporal artery-middle cerebral artery (STA-MCA) bypass, developed and popularized by Yasargil and Donaghy in the late 1960s [1], remains the most straightforward and versatile extracranial-intracranial (EC-IC) bypass method today, with applications in treating Moyamoya disease, cerebral aneurysms, and intracranial atherosclerosis.

Y. Liao · W. Ni · L. Chen · B. Xu (✉)
Huashan Hospital, Shanghai Medical College, Fudan University, Shanghai, China

3.2 Case 1

A 36-year-old man suffered from a sudden severe headache with nausea and vomiting 3 months prior. Physical examination did not reveal any neurological deficits. A head computed tomography (CT) scan 3 months ago demonstrated right caudate hemorrhage breaking into the bilateral ventricles (Fig. 3.1). After admission, digital subtraction angiography (DSA) showed Moyamoya disease, and the right external carotid artery (ECA) did not provide spontaneous compensation to the right hemisphere (Fig. 3.2). STA-MCA bypass with encephalo-duro-myo-synangiosis (EDMS) was planned for this patient (Fig. 3.3).

3.3 Details of the Procedure

During the operation, the patient was positioned supine in a headholder, and the head was rotated approximately 75° to the left side. An enlarged right pterional craniotomy was performed (Fig. 3.4). The skin incision was extended by 1.0–1.5 cm above the superior temporal line, and curved posteriorly as much as possible. The STA's posterior branch should be included in the flap for direct anastomosis (Fig. 3.5).

The temporal muscle was incised along the flap's posterior margin, then was dissected carefully from the temporal bone using a periosteal elevator without cautery. This maneuver exposed

Y. Mao et al. (eds.), *Surgical Atlas of Cerebral Revascularization*,
https://doi.org/10.1007/978-981-16-0374-7_3

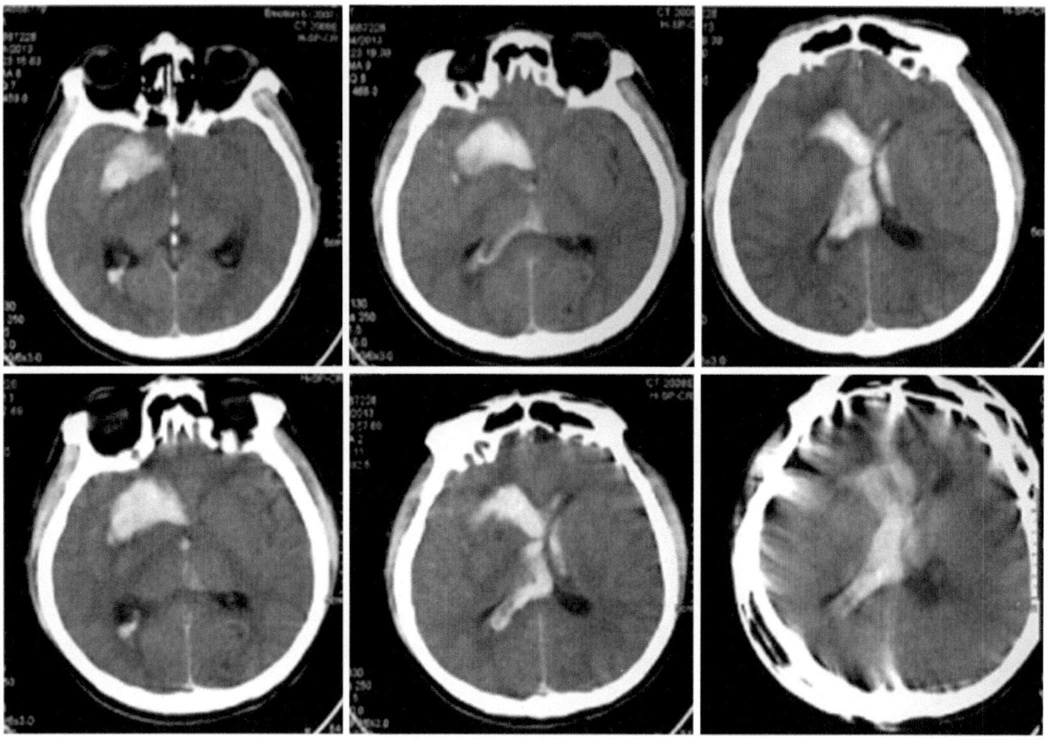

Fig. 3.1 Head CT scan 3 months ago demonstrated right caudate hemorrhage breaking into the bilateral ventricles

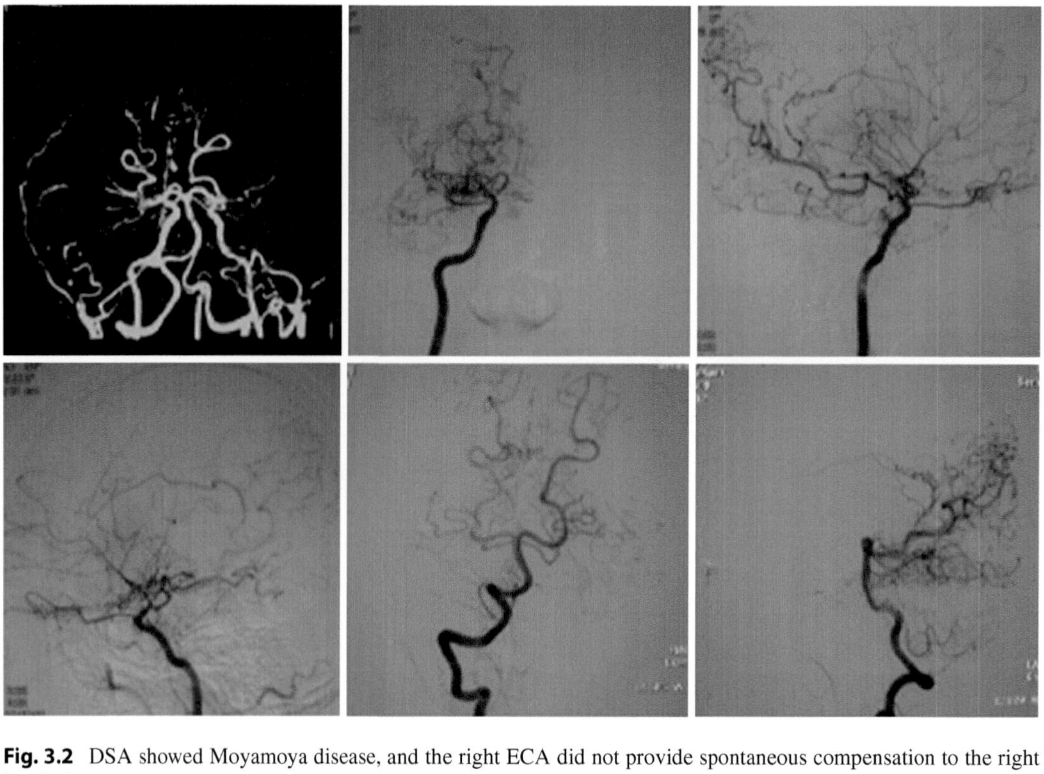

Fig. 3.2 DSA showed Moyamoya disease, and the right ECA did not provide spontaneous compensation to the right hemisphere

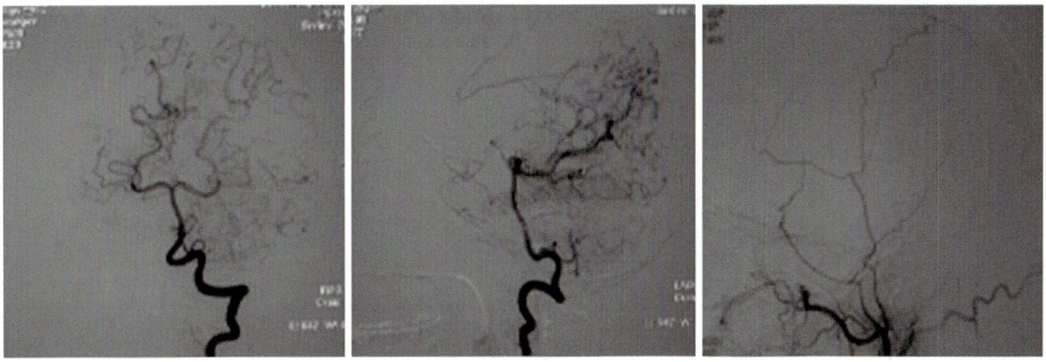

Fig. 3.2 (continued)

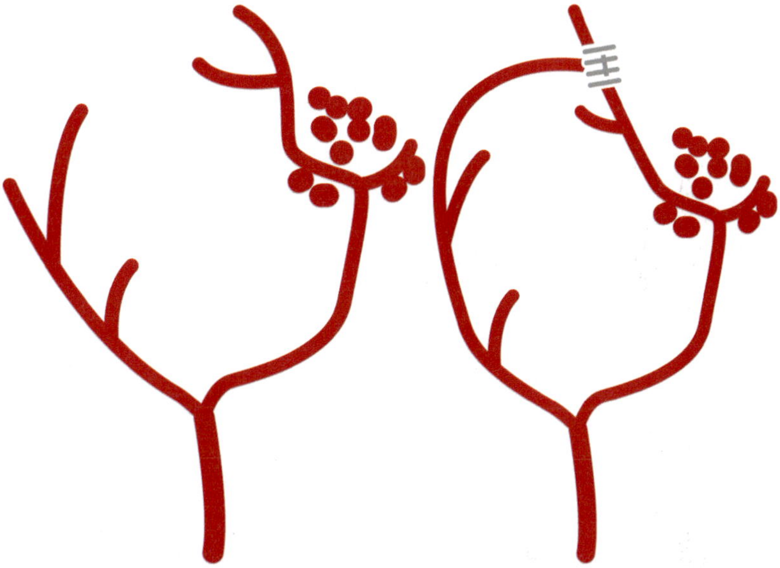

Fig. 3.3 Surgical plan: Right superficial temporal artery-middle cerebral artery (STA-MCA) bypass with encephalo-duro-myo-synangiosis (EDMS)

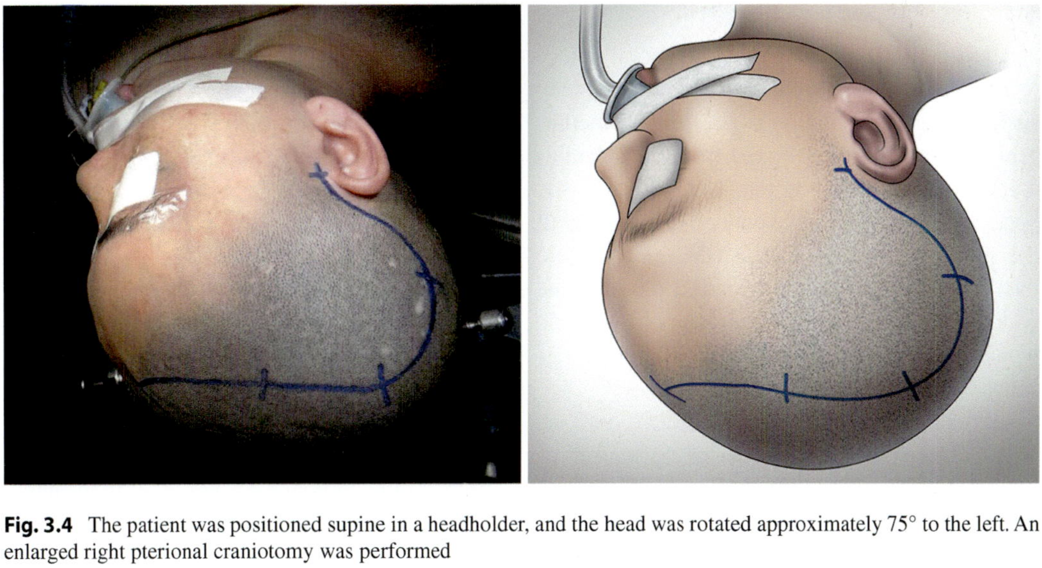

Fig. 3.4 The patient was positioned supine in a headholder, and the head was rotated approximately 75° to the left. An enlarged right pterional craniotomy was performed

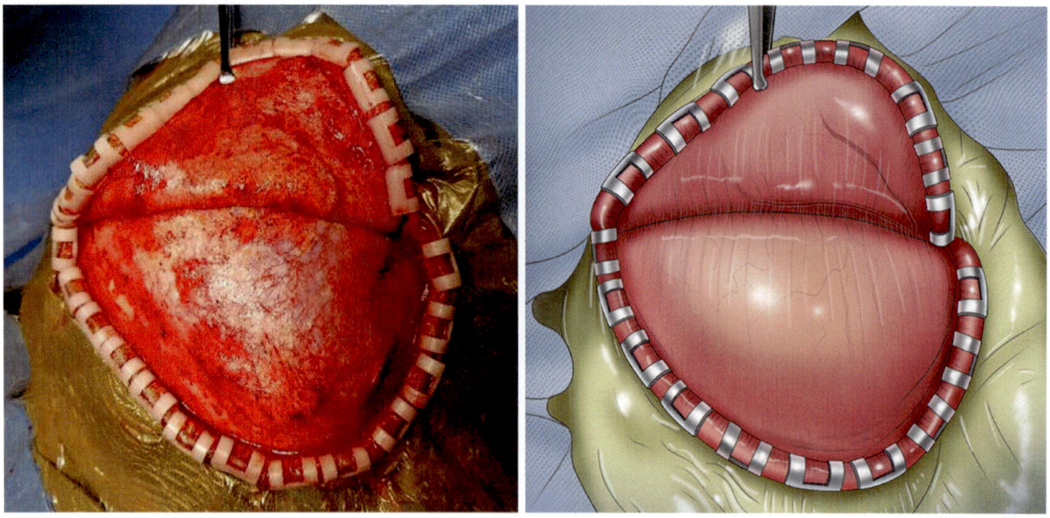

Fig. 3.5 The skin flap was dissected, and the STA branches were carefully preserved

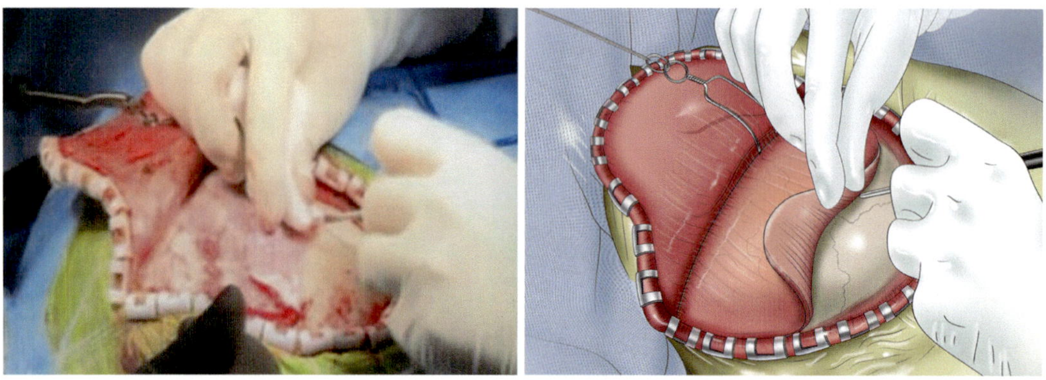

Fig. 3.6 The temporal muscle was incised from the bone using a periosteal elevator

and preserved the entire deep temporal artery (DTA) network on the temporal muscle's deep surface (Figs. 3.6 and 3.7). The middle meningeal artery (MMA) perforated from the sphenoidal crest. After the bone flap was removed, the bone window should be expanded carefully until this site without damaging the MMA. Holes were then drilled 2 cm along the edge of the bone window. The dura mater and temporal muscle would be fixed on them for EDMS after the STA-MCA bypass.

We then separated one branch of the STA. Monopolar electrical cautery was used to harvest the STA (Fig. 3.8). After penetrating the temporal muscle, the STA was pulled through (Figs. 3.9 and 3.10). The STA was then rinsed with pressurized heparin saline.

The dura mater on both sides of the sphenoidal crest residue was suspended and fixed. The avulsion or rupture of the MMA trunk should be avoided. To preserve MMA's main branches, the dura mater nearby should incise on both sides, resulting in strips with a width of 0.5–1.0 cm. The remaining dura mater were incised radially. After hemostasis, the dura mater was flipped over. The cranial surface of the dura mater could contact with the cortical surface closely (Fig. 3.11).

One of the cortical branches (M4) in the angular gyrus was selected as the recipient artery if it

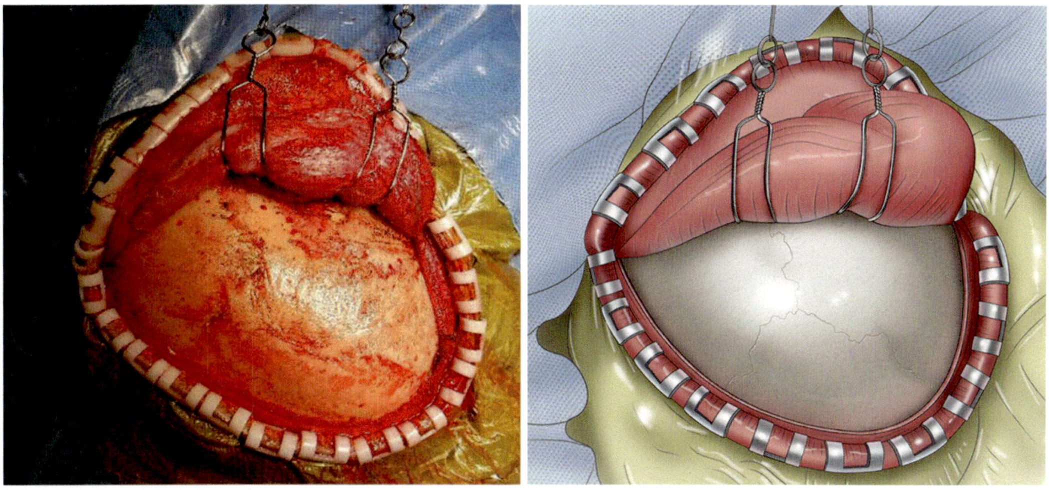

Fig. 3.7 The temporal muscle was dissected

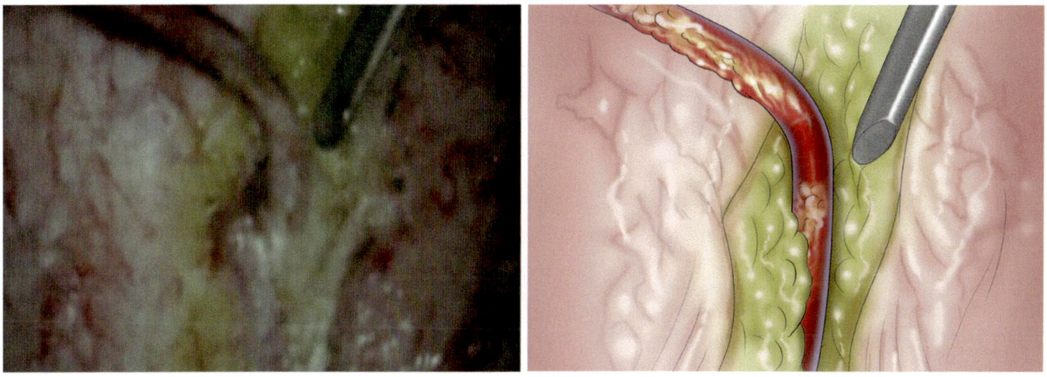

Fig. 3.8 One of the STA branches was detected subcutaneously in the skin flap. Monopolar electrical cautery was used to harvest the STA

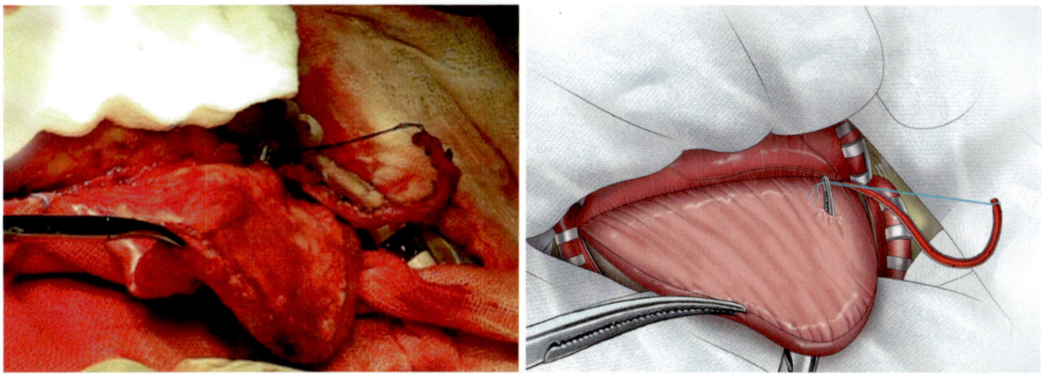

Fig. 3.9 After penetrating the temporal muscle, the STA was pulled through

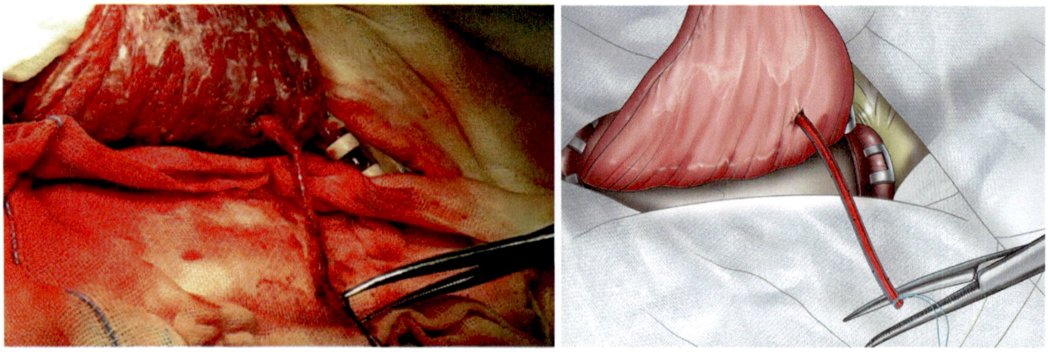

Fig. 3.10 The STA was pulled through the temporal muscle

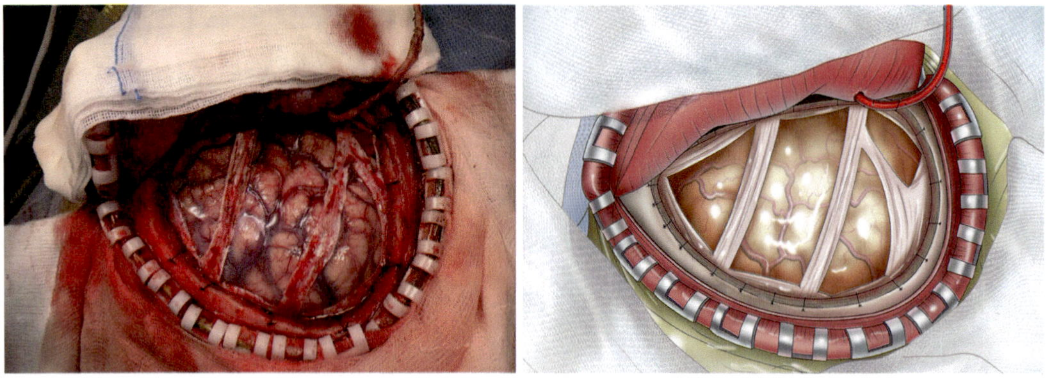

Fig. 3.11 After craniotomy, the dura mater was incised along each main branch of the MMA separately. The dura mater was flipped over and spread under the bone window with its cranial surface in close contact with the cortical surface

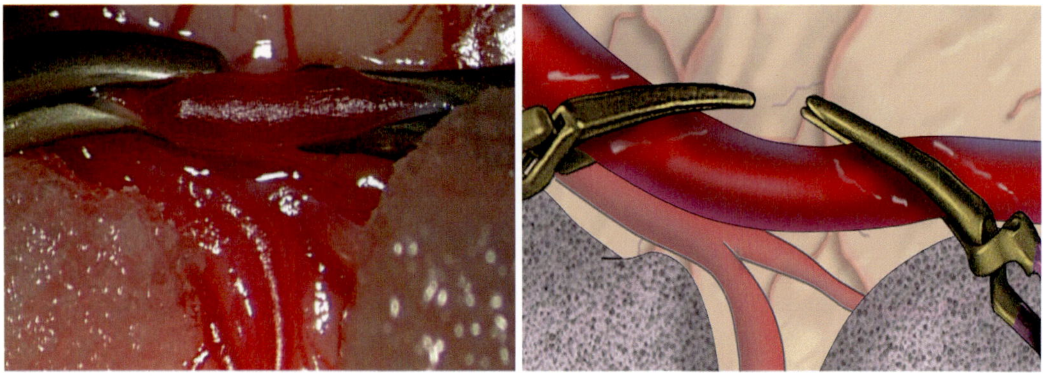

Fig. 3.12 One of the cortical branches (M4) in the angular gyrus was selected as the recipient artery if it was identical to the donor artery in size. This recipient artery was temporarily clipped for anastomosis

was identical to the donor artery in size. This recipient artery was temporarily clipped for anastomosis (Fig. 3.12). The divided STA branch was pulled to its vicinity and was then anastomosed with the recipient artery in an end-to-side fashion. We preferred a single 10.0 nylon atraumatic suture for anastomosis (Fig. 3.13). After anastomosis, the temporary clips on the recipient artery

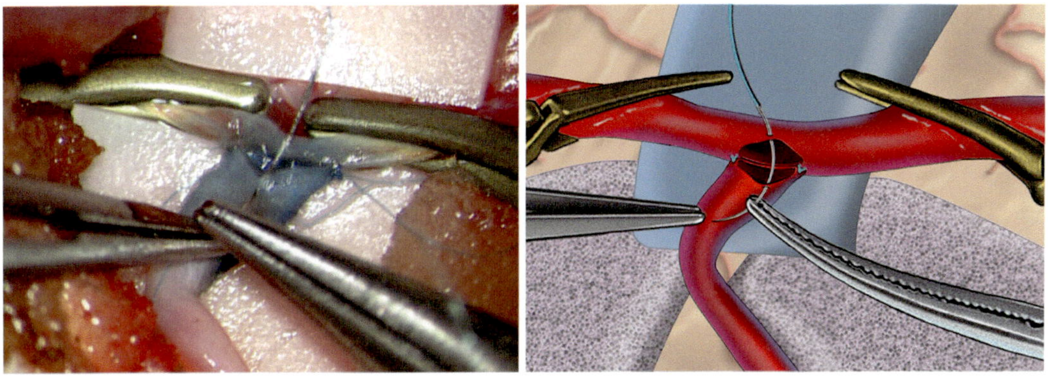

Fig. 3.13 An end-to-side anastomosis strategy was applied for the STA and the recipient M4 cortical branch for bypass

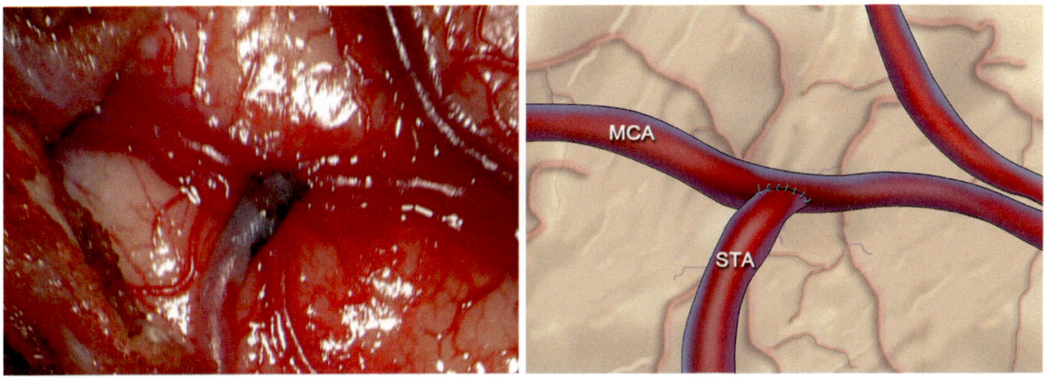

Fig. 3.14 After anastomosis, the temporary clips on the recipient artery were then removed to check for oozing from the anastomotic stoma, and additional stitches were placed to stop the bleeding, if necessary. If no oozing or stenosis of the anastomotic stoma were observed, the temporary clip on the root of the STA was removed

were then removed to check for oozing from the anastomotic stoma, and additional stitches could be placed to stop the bleeding, if necessary. If no oozing or stenosis of the anastomotic stoma was observed, the temporary clip on the root of the STA was removed (Fig. 3.14). After the anastomosis, indocyanine green (ICG) fluorescence angiography and Doppler ultrasound were applied to verify the anastomotic stoma's patency.

The temporal muscle margins were sutured with the flip-over dura mater at the fold and fixed to the bone window's edge (Fig. 3.15). The bone flap was trimmed and shaped compatibly, then fixed without STA compression. Because the positions of the temporal muscle and the bone flap were exchanged, the bone flap's inferior edge should be slightly elevated. This maneuver reduced the compression to the temporal muscle and might keep a good cosmetic appearance of the patient.

Postoperative DSA showed patency of the anastomosis and increased blood flow in the distal MCA (Fig. 3.16).

3.4 Case 2

A 49-year-old woman presented with episodic weakness of the bilateral limbs for 5 years. Physical examination did not reveal any neurological deficits. Head magnetic resonance imaging (MRI) demonstrated old infarction in the bilateral basal ganglion. Single-photon emission computed tomography (SPECT) showed hemispheric poor perfusion in the bilateral hemi-

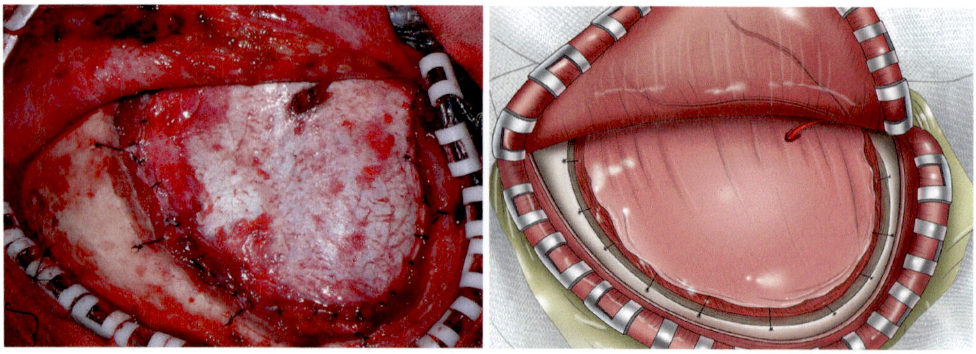

Fig. 3.15 The margins of the temporal muscle were fixed to the bone window. The bone flap was trimmed into a compatible shape and then fixed without compressing the STA

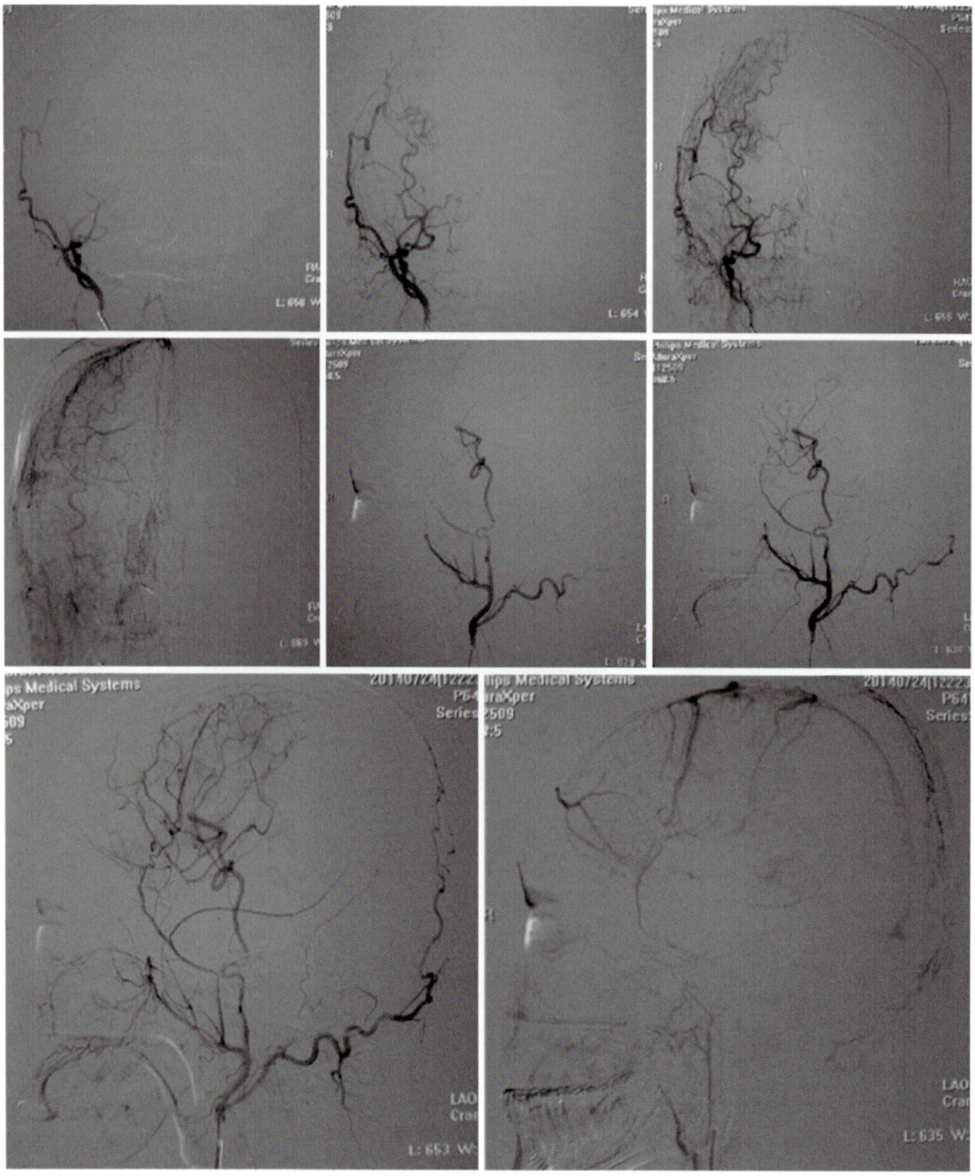

Fig. 3.16 Postoperative DSA showed patency of the anastomosis and increased blood flow in the distal MCA

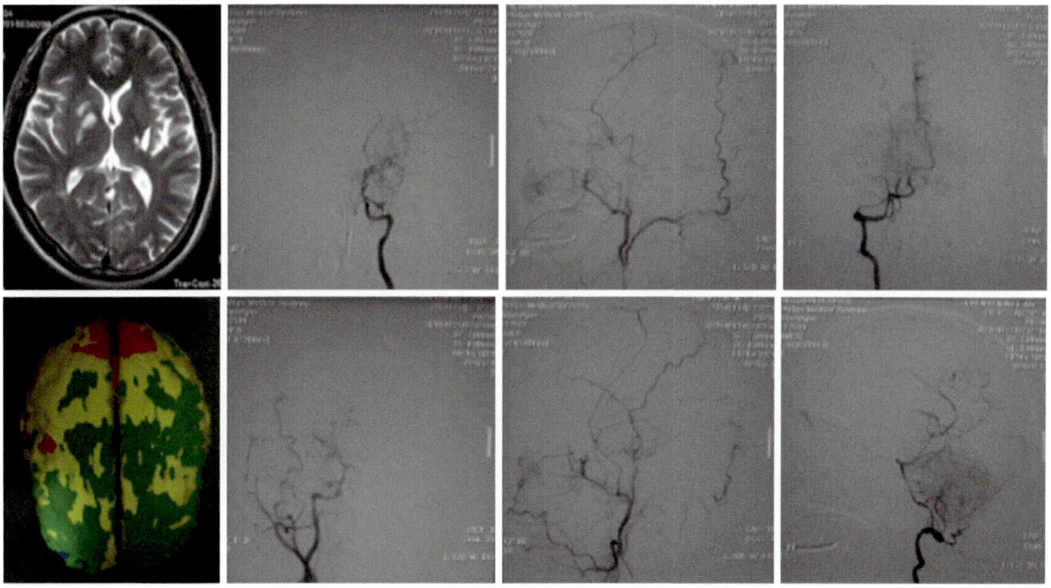

Fig. 3.17 Head MRI demonstrated old infarction in the bilateral basal ganglion. SPECT showed poor hemispheric perfusion in the bilateral hemispheres. DSA confirmed the diagnosis of Moyamoya disease, with some spontaneous collaterals from the MMA

Fig. 3.18 Surgical plan: STA-MCA double bypass with EDMS

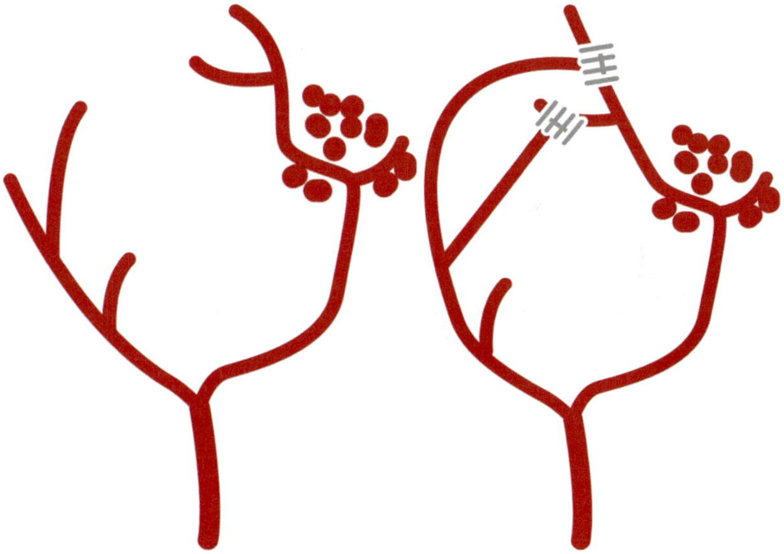

spheres. DSA confirmed the diagnosis of Moyamoya disease, with some spontaneous collaterals from the MMA (Fig. 3.17). Due to the severe hemispheric ischemia, an STA-MCA double bypass with EDMS was planned for this patient (Fig. 3.18). The right-sided surgery was performed first.

3.5 Details of the Procedure

During the operation, the patient was positioned supine, and the head was rotated approximately 75° to the left. An enlarged right pterional craniotomy was performed (Fig. 3.19). The skin incision was curved posteriorly, and both the ante-

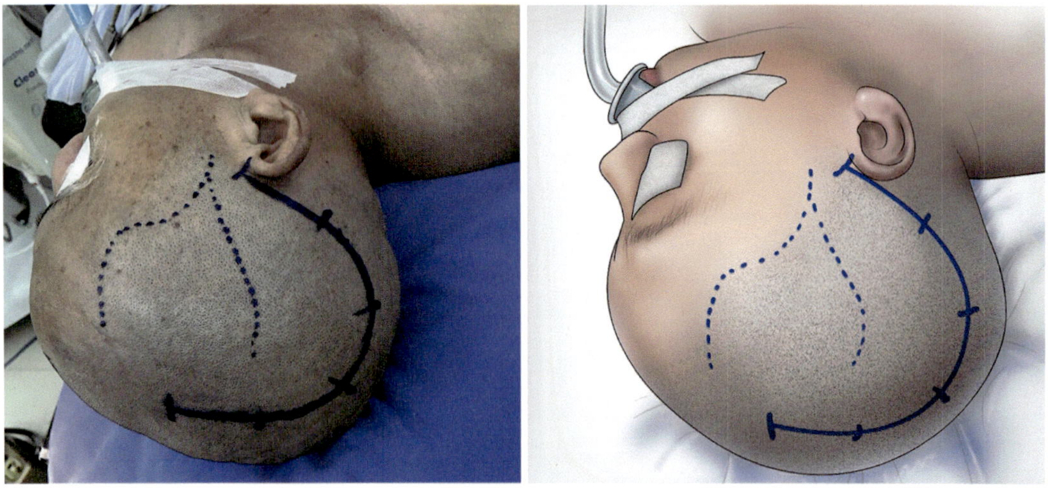

Fig. 3.19 The patient was positioned supine, and the head was rotated approximately 75° to the left. An enlarged right pterional craniotomy was performed

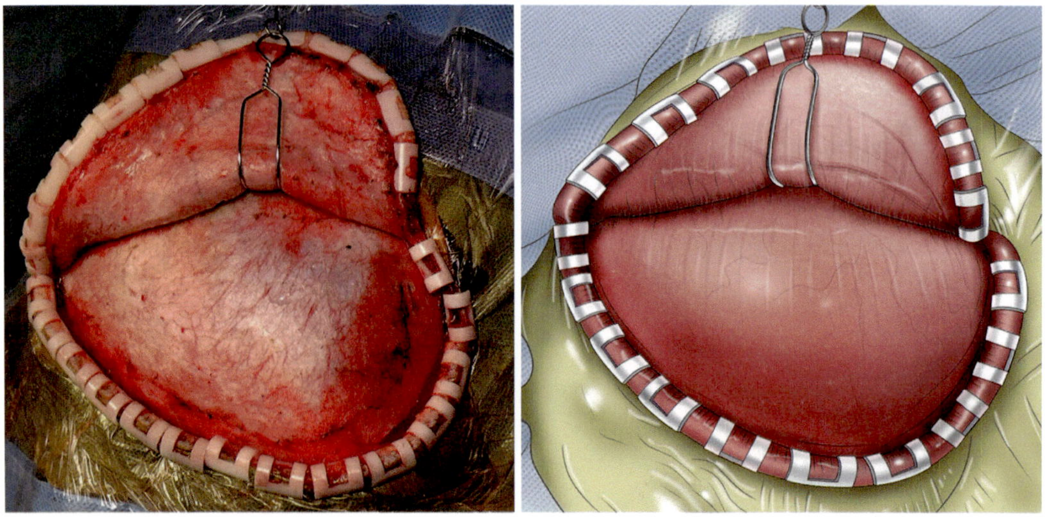

Fig. 3.20 The skin flap was dissected, and the STA branches were carefully preserved

rior (frontal) and the posterior (parietal) branches of the STA were carefully preserved (Fig. 3.20).

The temporal muscle was incised along the flap's posterior margin, then was dissected carefully from the temporal bone using a periosteal elevator without cautery (Fig. 3.21). The middle meningeal artery (MMA) perforated from the sphenoidal crest. After the bone flap was removed, the bone window should be expanded carefully until this site without damaging the MMA (Fig. 3.22). Holes were then drilled 2 cm along the edge of the bone window. Monopolar electrical cautery was used to harvest both the anterior (frontal) and posterior (parietal) branches of the STA. After penetrating the temporal muscle, both STA branches were pulled through, then rinsed with pressurized heparin saline (Fig. 3.23).

The dura mater on both sides of the sphenoidal crest residue was suspended and fixed. The avulsion or rupture of the MMA trunk should be avoided. To preserve the main branches of MMA, the dura mater should incise on both sides, result-

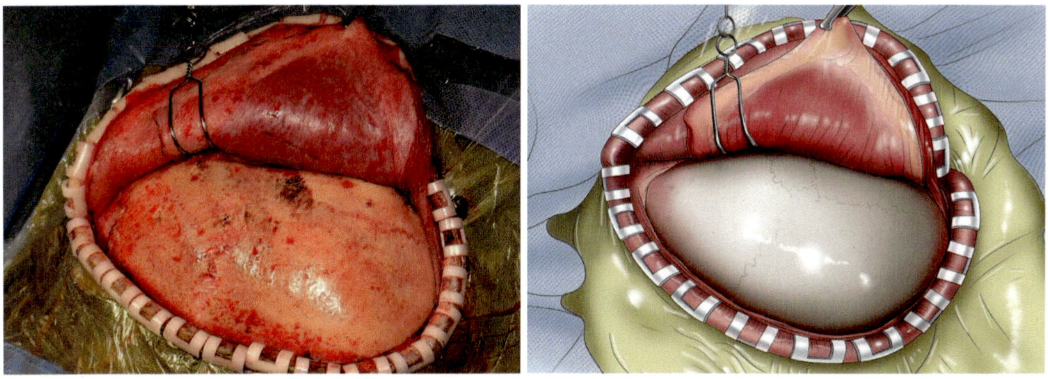

Fig. 3.21 The temporal muscle was dissected

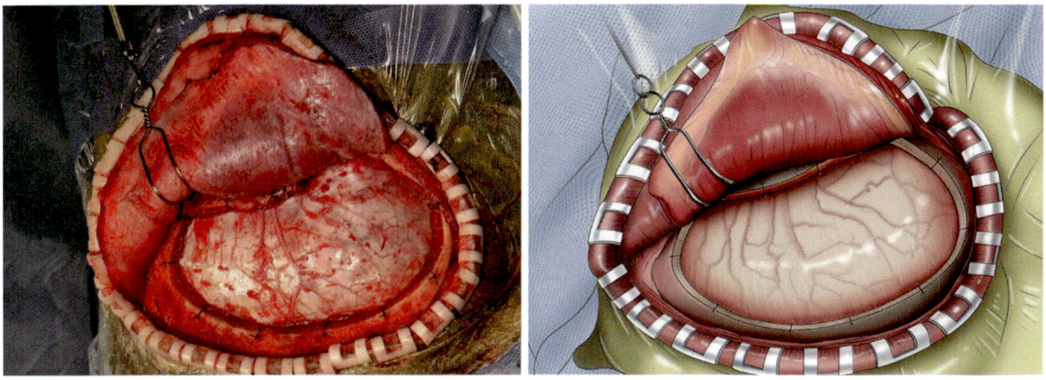

Fig. 3.22 The frontotemporal bone flap was elevated; the key step was to preserve the MMA

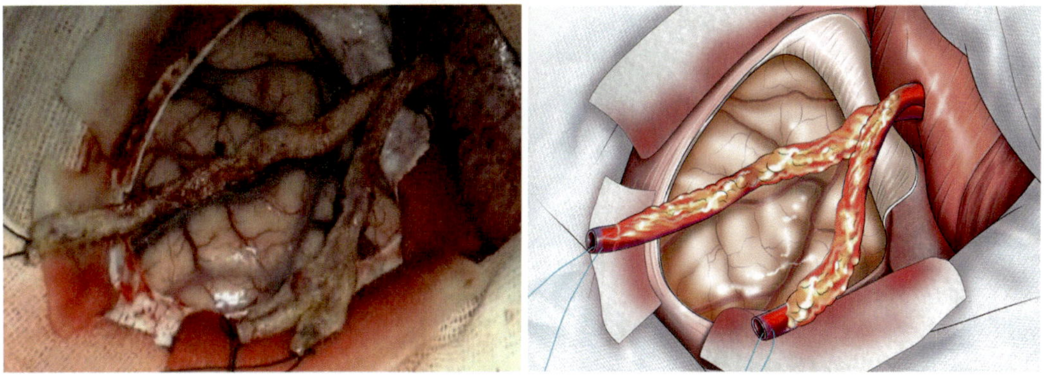

Fig. 3.23 Both STA branches penetrated through the temporal muscle

ing in strips with a width of 0.5–1.0 cm. The remaining dura mater was incised radially. After hemostasis, the dura mater was flipped over. The cranial surface of the dura mater could contact with the cortical surface closely.

Two of the cortical branches (M4) were selected as recipient arteries if identical to the donor artery in size. Both STA branches were anastomosed with the recipient arteries in an end-to-side fashion (Figs. 3.24–3.26). Indocyanine

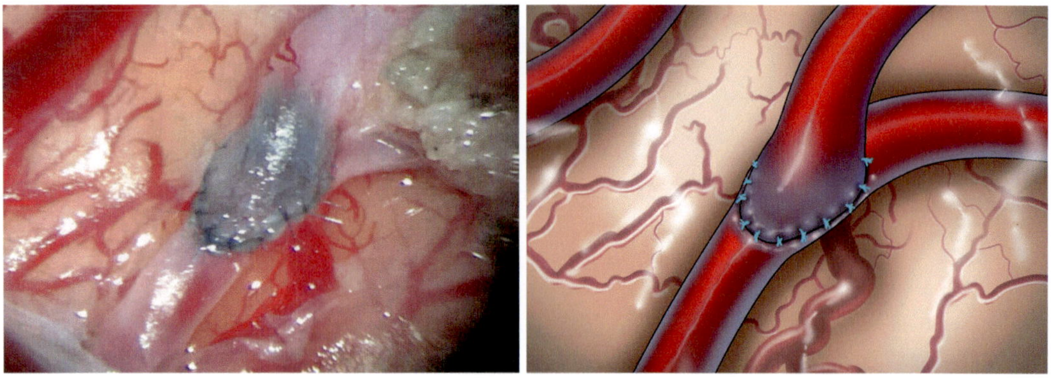

Fig. 3.24 The anterior (frontal) branch of the STA was anastomosed to one cortical MCA

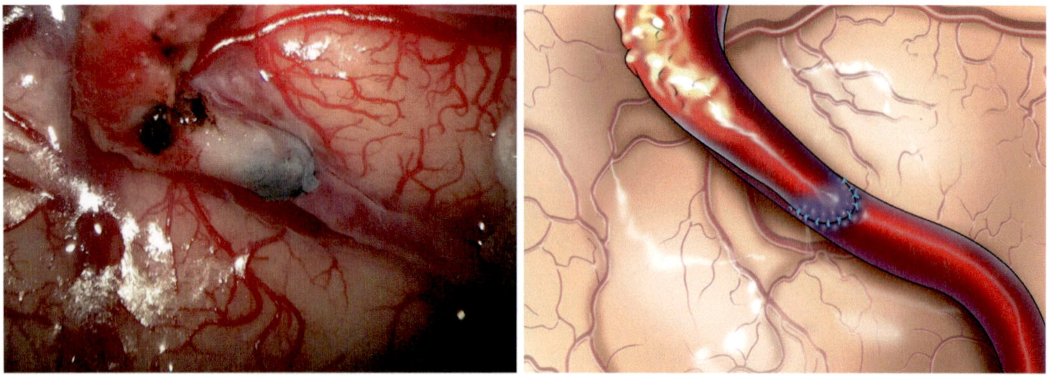

Fig. 3.25 The posterior (parietal) branch of the STA was anastomosed to another cortical MCA

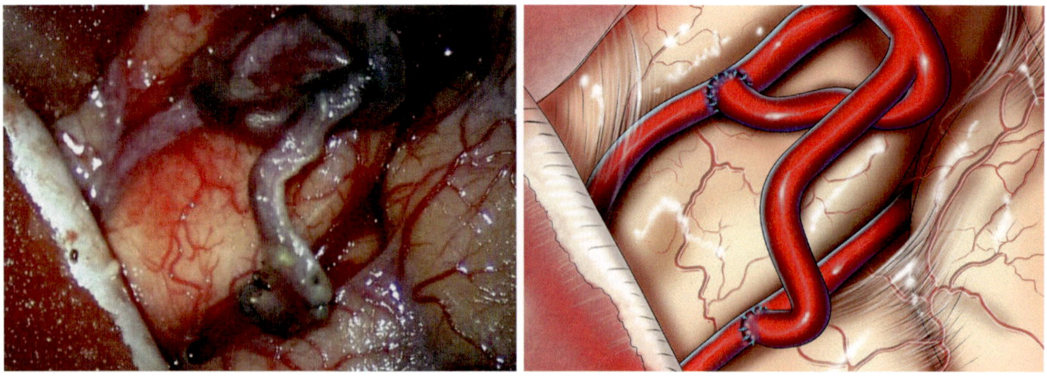

Fig. 3.26 A double STA-MCA bypass was completed

green (ICG) fluorescence angiography and Doppler ultrasound were applied to verify the bypass patency.

The temporal muscle margins were sutured with the flip-over dura mater at the fold and fixed to the bone window's edge. The bone flap was trimmed and shaped compatibly, then fixed without STA compression.

Postoperative DSA showed the patency of both anastomotic stomas (Fig. 3.27).

3.6 Case 3

A 21-year-old man underwent a right MCA aneurysm clipping 2 years ago and recently presented with seizure attacks. Physical examination did not reveal any neurological deficits. Computed tomography angiography (CTA) 2 years ago showed a right giant M1 aneurysm. The postoperative CTA showed no residual aneurysm after clipping. One year later, the follow-up CTA showed aneurysm recurrence (Fig. 3.28). The most recent CTA and preoperative DSA showed enlargement of the recurrent M1 aneurysm (Fig. 3.29). Because clipping a recurrent aneurysm is riskier, a protective STA-MCA bypass was planned before securing the aneurysm, and finally, the aneurysm was trapped with a patent bypass graft (Fig. 3.30).

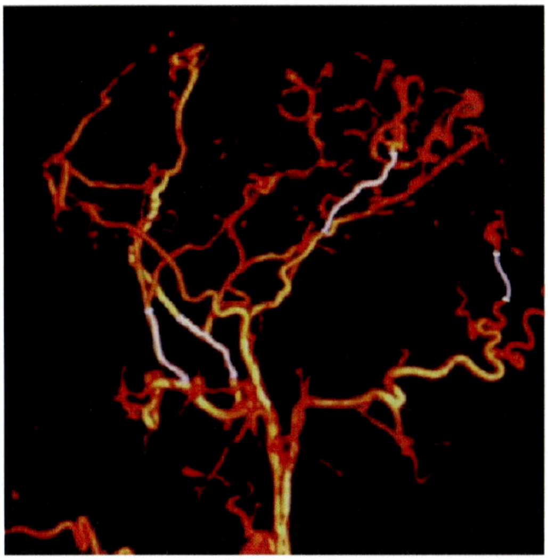

Fig. 3.27 Postoperative DSA indicated that both stomas were patent

3.7 Details of the Procedure

During the operation, the patient was positioned supine, and the head was rotated approximately 45° to the left. A right pterional craniotomy was performed. The Sylvian fissure was widely opened, and the frontal lobe was slightly retracted to expose the ipsilateral ICA. The previous aneurysm clip was stable, and no recurrence was observed on the proximal or distal end. There was a fusiform expansion of the M1

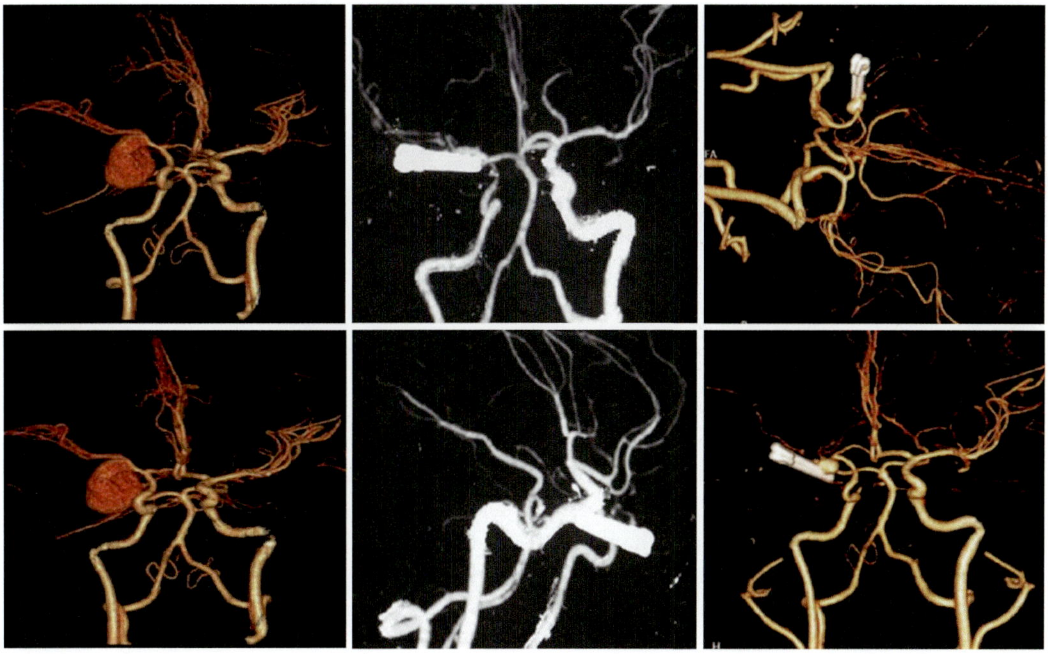

Fig. 3.28 CTA showed a right giant M1 aneurysm 2 years ago (left). The postoperative CTA showed no residual aneurysm after clipping (middle). One year later, the follow-up CTA showed aneurysm recurrence (right)

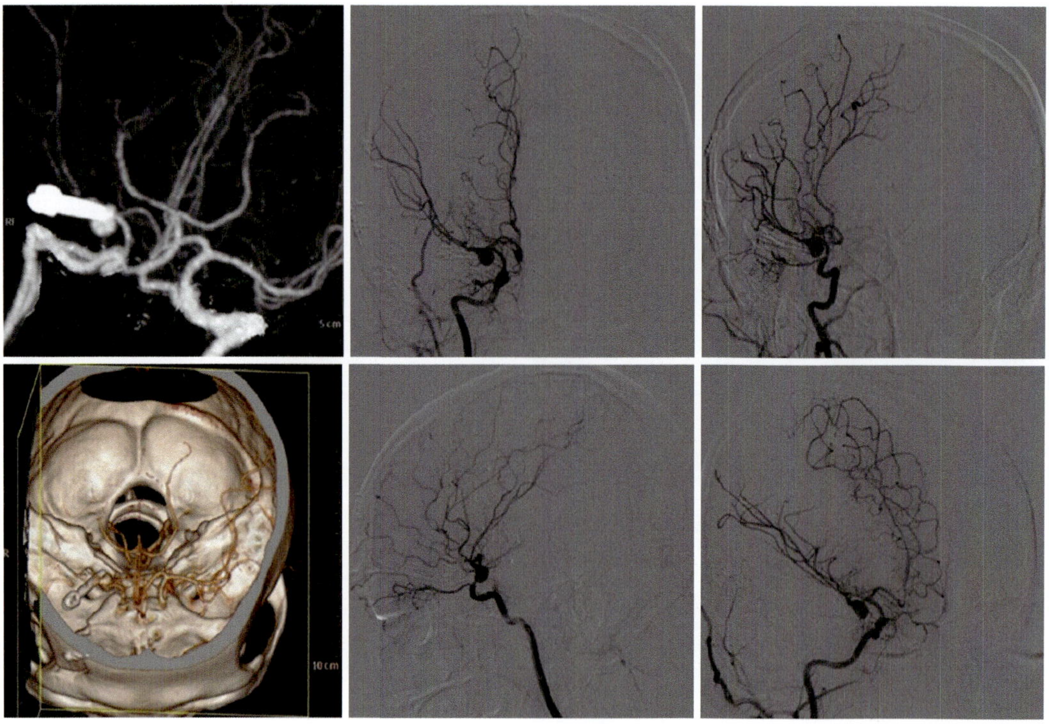

Fig. 3.29 The most recent CTA and preoperative DSA showed enlargement of the recurrent M1 aneurysm

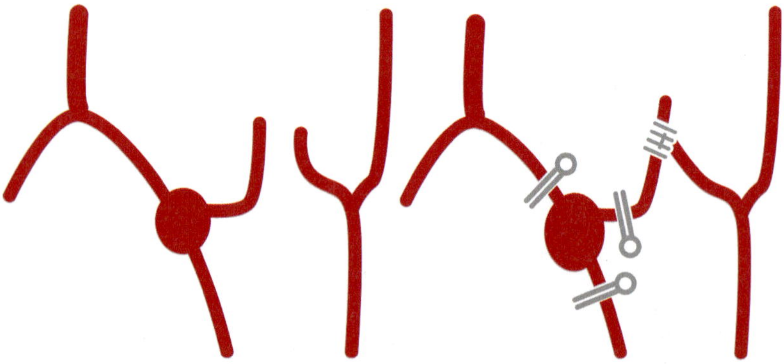

Fig. 3.30 A protective STA-MCA bypass was planned before securing the aneurysm, and finally, the aneurysm was trapped with a patent bypass graft

segment bulging mainly toward the temporal lobe (Fig. 3.31).

The severe intimal hyperplasia of the aneurysmal wall prevented direct aneurysm clipping due to arterial stiffness. Fortunately, the lenticulostriate perforators did not originate from the body of the aneurysm (Fig. 3.32). Therefore, we performed a STA-MCA protective bypass before securing the aneurysm. Because of the STA branch's sufficient length and size, we could anastomose the STA branch to the M3 to provide adequate cerebral blood flow perfusion without a graft. An end-to-side bypass was performed (Figs. 3.33 and 3.34). The aneurysm was then trapped, and all perforating arteries were spared (Fig. 3.35). The motor evoked potentials (MEPs) and somatosensory evoked potential (SEPs) were stable during the procedure for 2 h. The illustrated diagram demonstrates the treatment strategy (Fig. 3.36).

The patient recovered without any neurological deficits. The postoperative CTA demonstrated the patency of the bypass graft and complete obliteration of the aneurysm (Fig. 3.37).

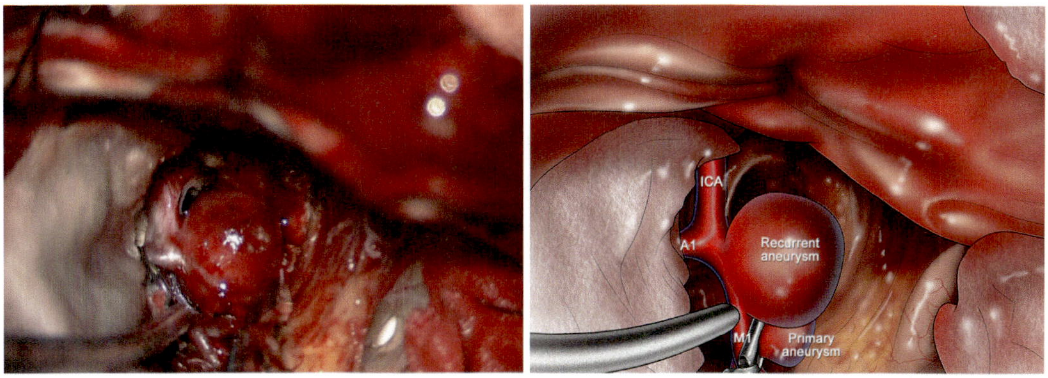

Fig. 3.31 The sylvian fissure was dissected, and the frontal lobe was slightly retracted to expose the ipsilateral ICA. The previous aneurysm clip was stable, and no recurrence was observed on the proximal or distal end. There was a fusiform expansion of the M1 segment bulging mainly toward the temporal lobe

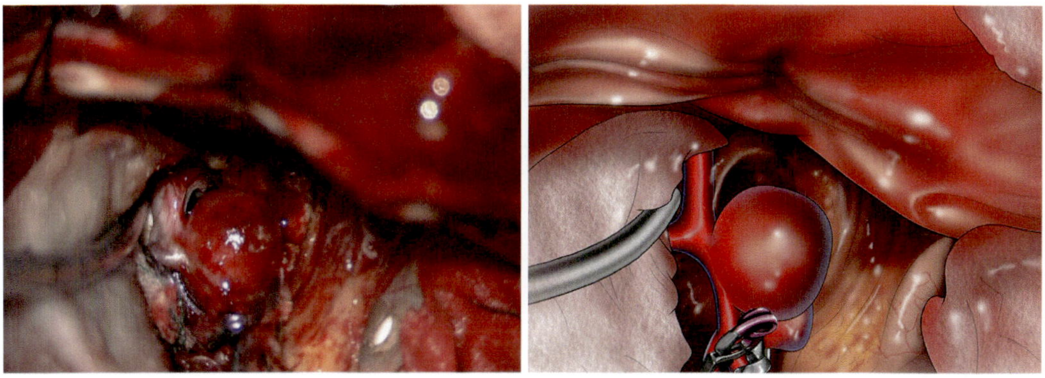

Fig. 3.32 Intraoperative findings showed an aneurysm with severe intimal hyperplasia of the aneurysmal wall. Fortunately, the lenticulostriate perforators did not originate from the site of the aneurysm

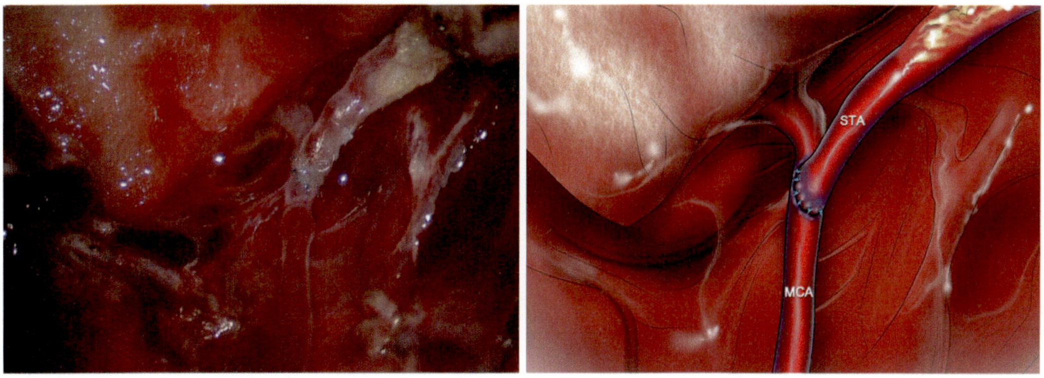

Fig. 3.33 STA–M3 bypass was performed in an end-to-side fashion

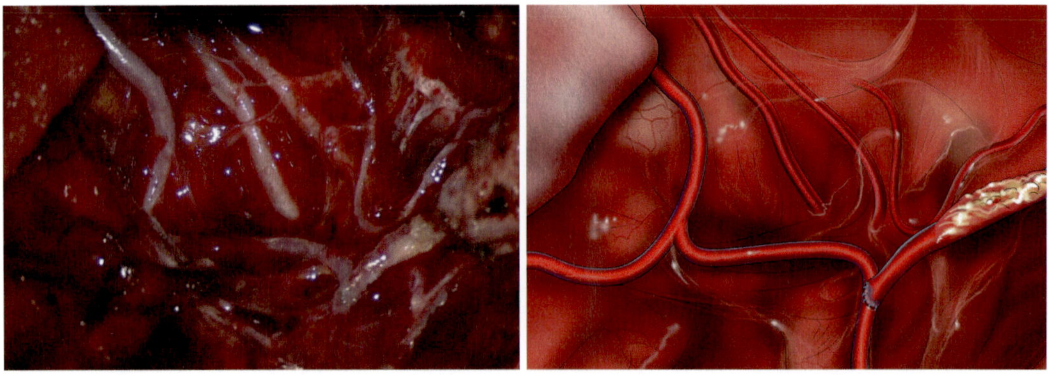

Fig. 3.34 After bypass was completed, the temporary clips were removed, and a Doppler ultrasound probe was utilized to ensure patency of the anastomosis

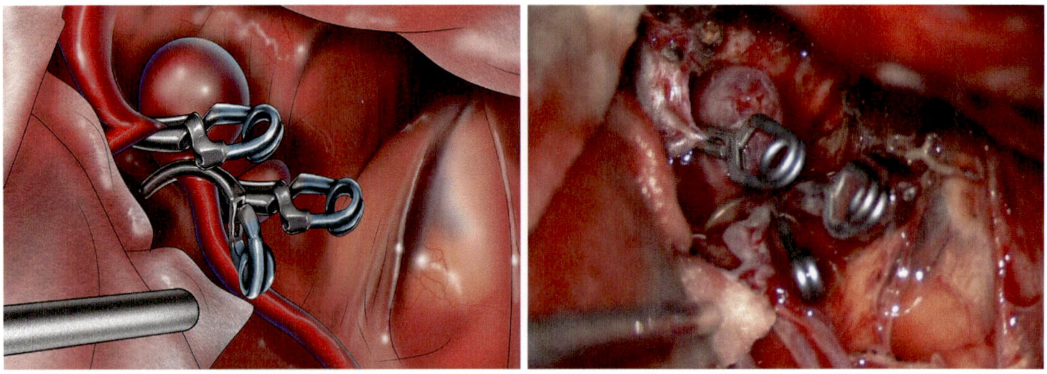

Fig. 3.35 The aneurysm was then trapped after STA–M3 bypass, and all perforating arteries were spared

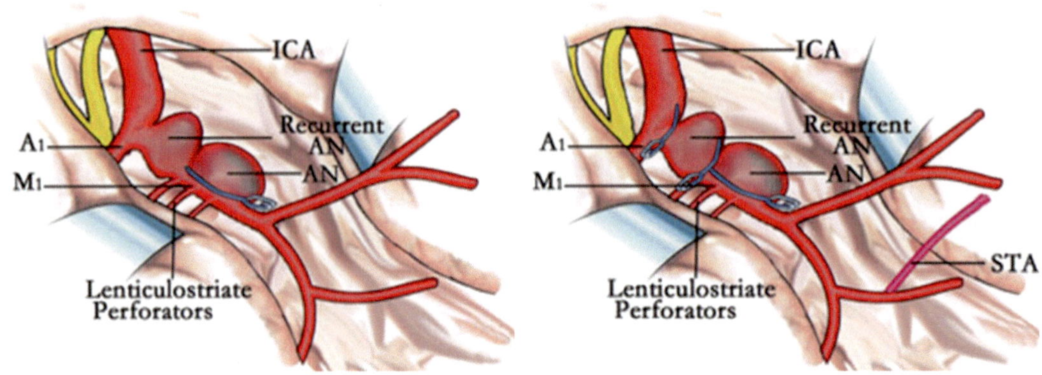

Fig. 3.36 The diagram of the intraoperative findings on the left shows the recurrent aneurysm originating from the proximal M1 segment. The diagram on the right shows that the recurrent aneurysm was trapped without injury to the lenticulostriate perforators (Reproduced from Zhu W, Liu P, Tian Y, Gu Y, Xu B, Chen L, Zhou L, Mao Y. Complex middle cerebral artery aneurysms: a new classification based on the angioarchitecture and surgical strategies. Acta Neurochir. 2013; 155(8): 1481–91.)

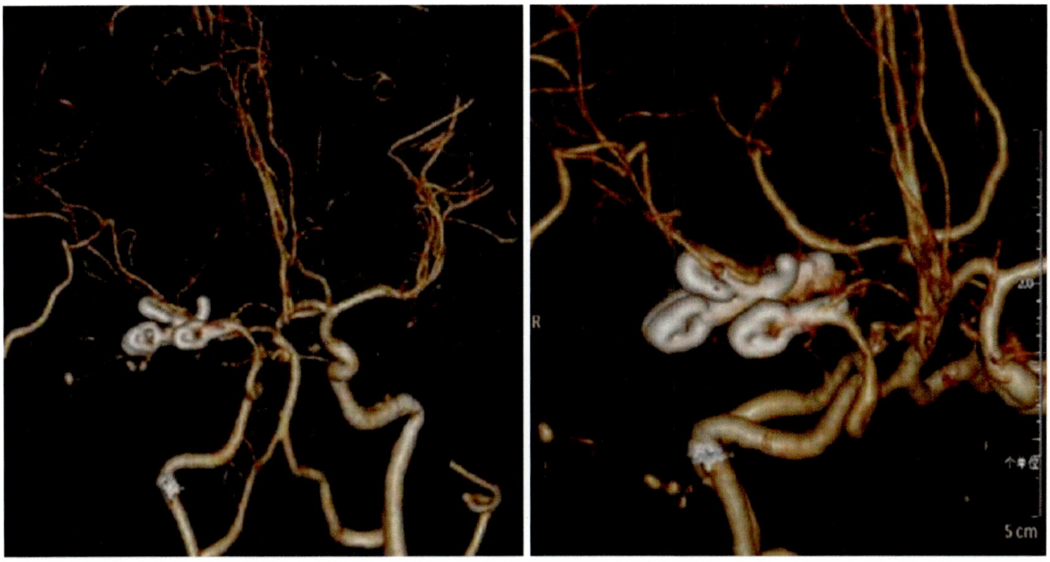

Fig. 3.37 Postoperative CTA demonstrated complete obliteration of the aneurysm and patency of the bypass graft

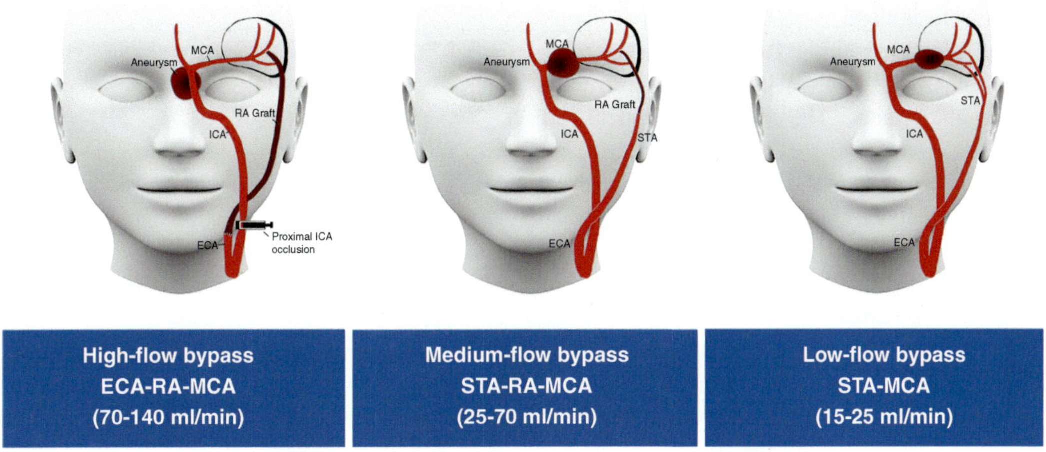

Fig. 3.38 The EC-IC bypass technique can be classified as high-flow (ECA-RA-MCA), medium-flow (STA-RA-MCA), and low-flow (STA-MCA) bypass, providing different blood flow volumes

3.8 Comment

In our experience, the EC-IC bypass technique can be classified as high-flow (ECA-RA-MCA), medium-flow (STA-RA-MCA), and low-flow (STA-MCA) bypass, providing different blood flow volumes (Fig. 3.38). STA-MCA bypass is the most commonly used low-flow EC-IC bypass technique for cerebral vascular disease affecting the anterior circulation, but the procedure is slightly different for the surgical treatment of Moyamoya disease and complex aneurysms [2, 3].

3.8.1 Moyamoya Disease

Surgical management for Moyamoya disease includes direct and indirect revascularizations. Three types of ECA branches are involved in these procedures: (1) the STA or the occipital artery supplying the scalp and galea aponeurotica. They could be anastomosed to the intracranial cortical arteries for direct bypass; (2) the DTA supplying the periosteum and temporal muscle. The sphenopalatine artery might also contribute to the supply of the anterior part of the temporal muscle in some cases; and (3) the MMA supplying the dura mater [4, 5]. As illustrated in cases 1 and 2, we advocated for indirect revascularization, termed EDMS, for Moyamoya disease surgery in addition to the direct bypass [4, 5]. The EDMS achieved maximal use of the MMA and DTA, and promoted spontaneous anastomosis 3 or 4 months postoperatively [6].

Therefore, the DTA and the MMA network's integrity and the pre-existing spontaneous anastomoses from them to the cortical arteries should be well preserved during craniotomy. Preoperative assessment of the MMA localization is of paramount importance. The MMA's cranial groove could be observed on the DSA mask images. The relationship between the MMA groove and coronal suture helps localize the MMA during craniotomy. Normally, the MMA course is approximately parallel to that of the STA parietal branch, approximately 2–3 cm anteriorly. If the MMA groove seemed shallow and vague on the DSA mask images, we performed a single-window heart-shaped craniotomy and expanded the bone window toward the sphenoidal crest to the site where the MMA perforated. However, if the MMA groove was deep and clear on the DSA mask images, we preferred double-window bone flaps anterior and posterior to the MMA. We left a bone bridge to cover the course of the MMA. For the DTA network preservation, we avoided excessive temporal muscle cautery. The temporal muscle was bluntly dissected carefully from the bone to keep the entire DTA network intact [4, 5].

Neurosurgeons should also recognize the pre-existing spontaneous collaterals on angiography very carefully before surgery and perform individualized craniotomy and bypass. Spontaneous collaterals in Moyamoya disease create some normally perfused islands in the ischemic hemisphere. Furthermore, the ECA cannot completely replace the ICA due to anatomical restrictions. On the basis of these two facts, target revascularization is reasonable and may facilitate blood flow to where it is mostly demanded; in some circumstances, multiple bypasses were necessary, even when there was only one single STA available for direct bypass; in this case, two donor arteries were created. The ischemic area could be defined by hemodynamic evaluation with CTP or SPECT. The scalp flap and bone window should cover this area as much as possible in the surgical plan. The totally infarcted area should be avoided, as revascularization would not be useful. The normally perfused island should not be the target area because it has a lower blood flow requirement than the ischemic area.

3.8.2 Complex Intracranial Aneurysm

For complex aneurysm surgery, low-flow STA-MCA bypass is mainly used as a protective or flow-diverting revascularization technique. The length of the dissected STA in this case should be longer than that in surgeries for Moyamoya disease because the vessel is usually anastomosed to the M3 segment inside the Sylvian fissure for proximal MCA aneurysms, and this segment is deeper than the cortical MCA branches, as seen in case 3 [3]. For distal MCA aneurysms, IC-IC bypass is usually preferred instead of EC-IC bypass.

References

1. Donaghy RM, Yasargil G. Microangeional surgery and its techniques. Prog Brain Res. 1968;30:263–7.
2. Hori S, Kashiwazaki D, Akioka N, Hayashi T, Hori E, Umemura K, Horie Y, Kuroda S. Surgical anatomy and preservation of the middle meningeal artery during bypass surgery for moyamoya disease. Acta Neurochir. 2015;157(1):29–36.

3. Zhu W, Liu P, Tian Y, Gu Y, Xu B, Chen L, Zhou L, Mao Y. Complex middle cerebral artery aneurysms: a new classification based on the angioarchitecture and surgical strategies. Acta Neurochir. 2013;155(8):1481–91.
4. Xu B, Song DL, Mao Y, Gu YX, Xu H, Liao YJ, Liu CH, Zhou LF. Superficial temporal artery-middle cerebral artery bypass combined with encephalo-duro-myo-synangiosis in treating moyamoya disease: surgical techniques, indications and midterm follow-up results. Chin Med J. 2012;125(24):4398–405.
5. Shen W, Xu B, Li H, Gao X, Liao Y, Shi W, Zhao R, Zhang Y. Enlarged encephalo-duro-myo-synangiosis treatment for moyamoya disease in young children. World Neurosurg. 2017;106:9–16.
6. Houkin K, Nakayama N, Kuroda S, Ishikawa T, Nonaka T. How does angiogenesis develop in pediatric moyamoya disease after surgery? A prospective study with MR angiography. Childs Nerv Syst. 2004;20(10):734–41.

4 Middle Cerebral Artery-Middle Cerebral Artery Bypass

Zixiao Yang and Wei Zhu

Abstract

In this in situ bypass technique, a side-to-side anastomosis of the arteries distal and adjacent to the aneurysm is achieved. The advantages of this method include avoiding the radial artery as the donor artery and subsequent cervical incision, achieving complete restoration of the skull bone flap, and obtaining a similar diameter between the donor and recipient arteries. This procedure is suitable for treating large or giant middle cerebral artery (MCA) aneurysms that are not viable for coiling or clipping.

Keywords

Intracranial aneurysm · Intracranial-intracranial bypass · In situ bypass · Middle cerebral artery · Revascularization

4.1 Introduction

In this in situ bypass technique, a side-to-side anastomosis of the arteries distal and adjacent to the aneurysm is achieved. The advantages of this method include avoiding the radial artery as the donor artery and subsequent cervical incision, achieving complete restoration of the skull bone flap, and obtaining a similar diameter between the donor and recipient arteries. This procedure is suitable for treating large or giant middle cerebral artery (MCA) aneurysms that are not viable for coiling or clipping [1].

4.2 Case

A 55-year-old man presented with headache for 6 months. Physical examination did not reveal any neurological deficits. Head computed tomography (CT), magnetic resonance imaging (MRI), and digital subtraction angiography (DSA) demonstrated a large left MCA (M2) dissecting aneurysm, with obvious calcification on the aneurysm body (Fig. 4.1). Endovascular treatment was not suitable for this patient, and direct clipping was also impossible. Therefore, to secure the aneurysm, a left side-to-side MCA-MCA bypass combined with aneurysm trapping was planned (Fig. 4.2).

4.3 Details of the Procedure

During the operation, the patient was positioned supine with the head turned 60° to the right, and the left shoulder was elevated. The head was elevated by 20 degrees to facilitate venous drainage. A modified pterional craniotomy was applied,

Z. Yang · W. Zhu (✉)
Huashan Hospital, Shanghai Medical College, Fudan University, Shanghai, China
e-mail: drzhuwei@fudan.edu.cn

Y. Mao et al. (eds.), *Surgical Atlas of Cerebral Revascularization*,
https://doi.org/10.1007/978-981-16-0374-7_4

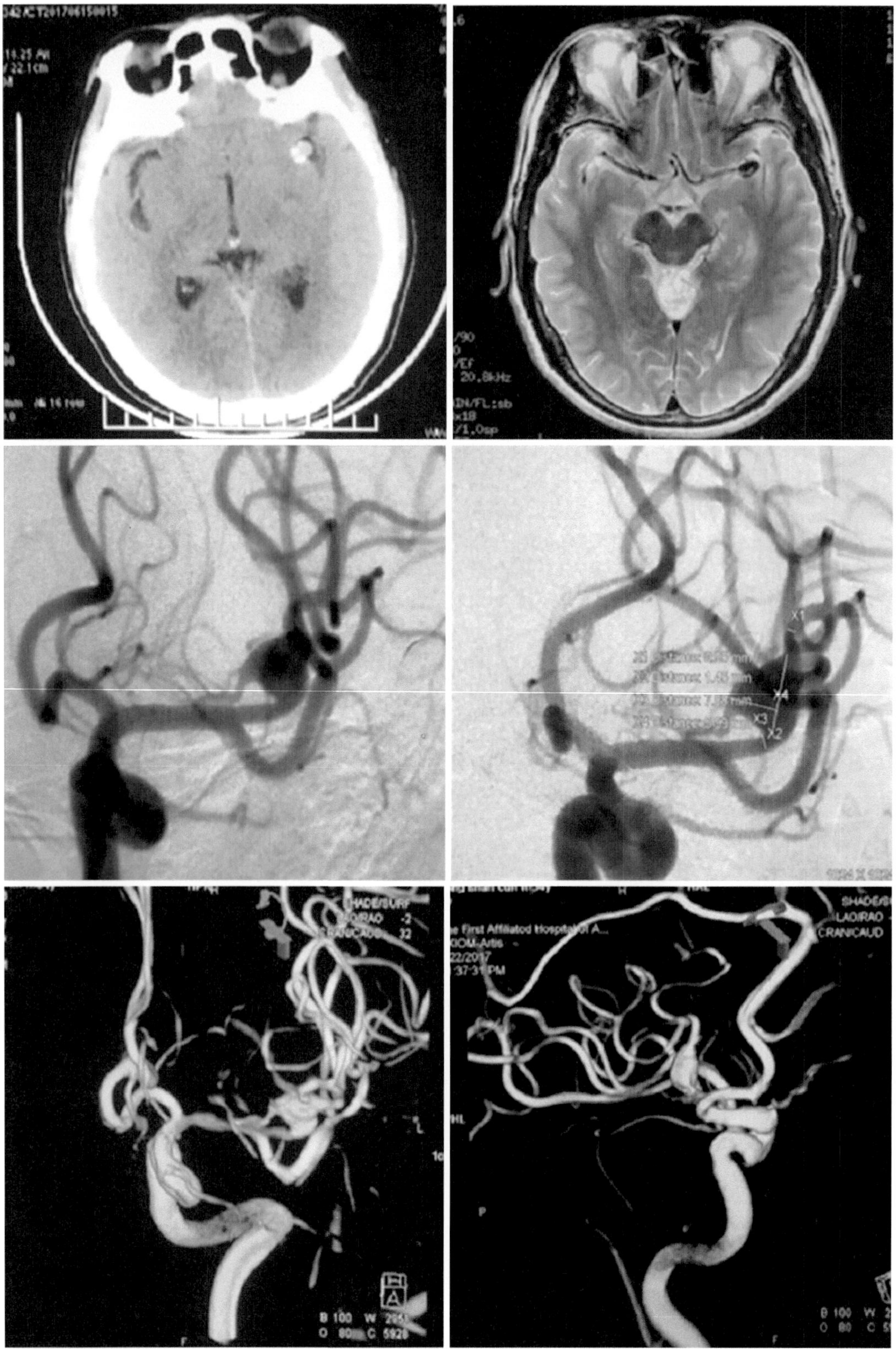

Fig. 4.1 Head CT, MRI, and DSA demonstrated a large left MCA (M2) dissecting aneurysm, with obvious calcification on the aneurysm body

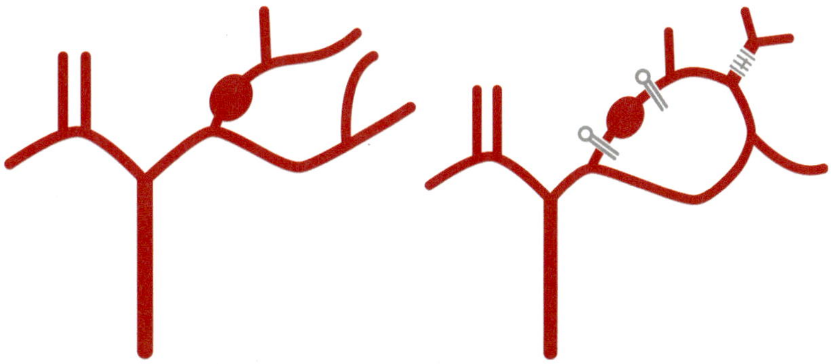

Fig. 4.2 Surgical plan: left side-to-side MCA-MCA bypass combined with aneurysm trapping

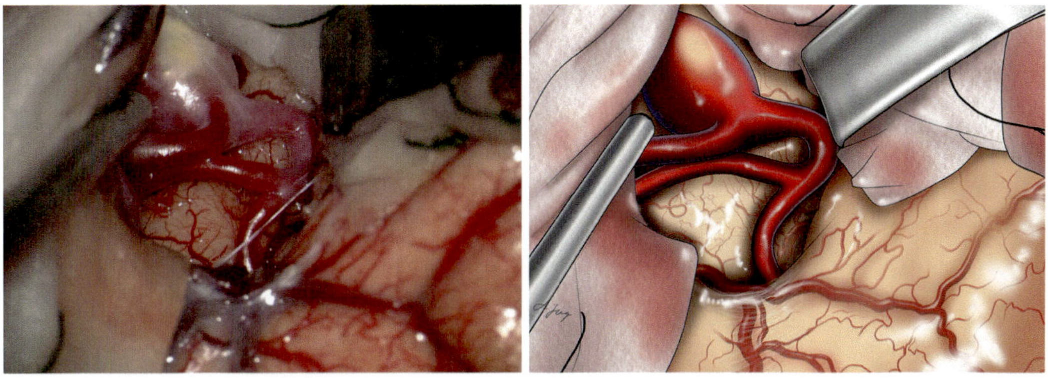

Fig. 4.3 A modified pterional craniotomy was applied, and the sylvian fissure was dissected under a microscope to expose the aneurysm and MCA branches

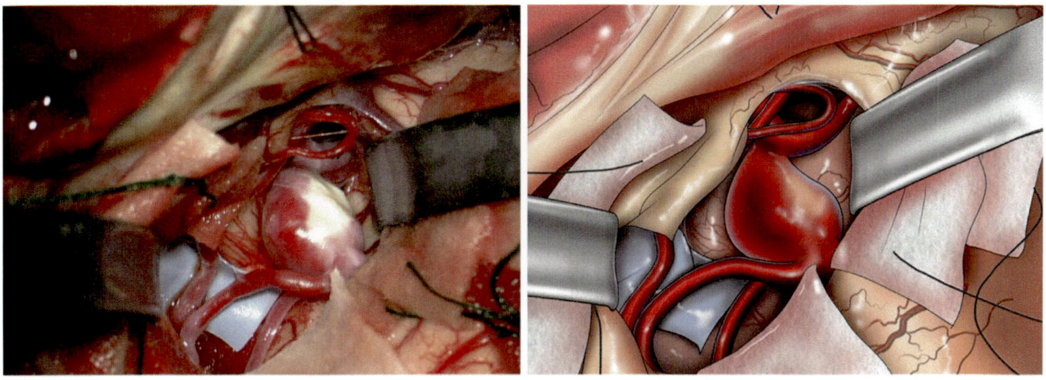

Fig. 4.4 The aneurysm was located in the M2 frontal branch and a perforating artery originating from the proximal portion of the aneurysm

and the sylvian fissure was dissected under a microscope to expose the aneurysm and MCA branches (Fig. 4.3). The aneurysm was located in the M2 frontal branch and a perforating artery originating from the proximal portion of the aneurysm (Fig. 4.4).

With no aneurysms present in the M2 temporal branch, side-to-side suturing of the temporal and frontal M2 arteries was planned to achieve anastomosis (Fig. 4.5). The temporal and frontal M2 branches were occluded temporarily to determine a suitable location and length of the poten-

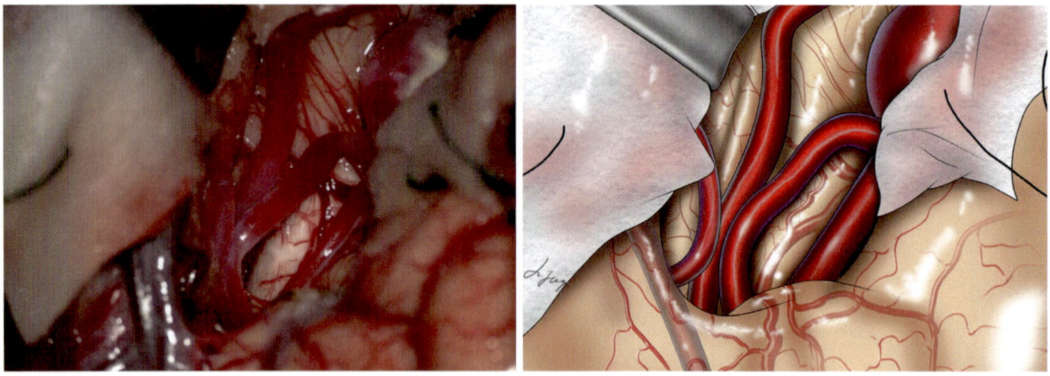

Fig. 4.5 With no aneurysms present in the M2 temporal branch, side-to-side suturing of the temporal and frontal M2 arteries was planned to achieve anastomosis

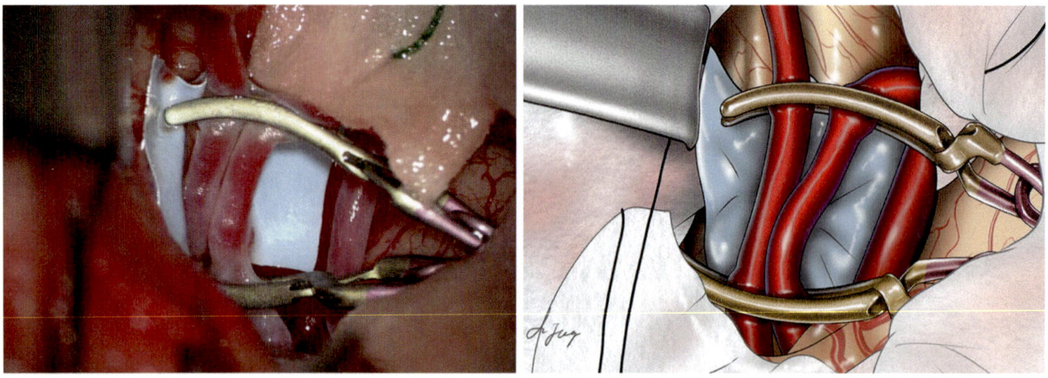

Fig. 4.6 The temporal and frontal M2 branches were occluded temporarily to determine a suitable location and length of the potential anastomosis

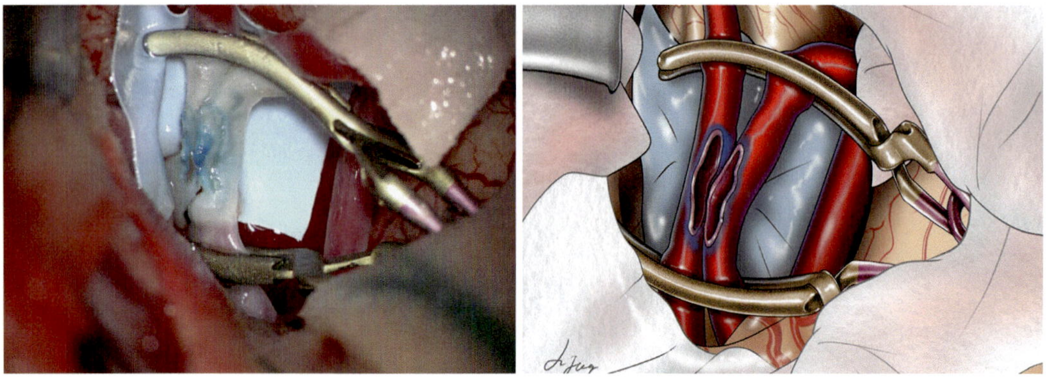

Fig. 4.7 Linear arteriotomy was performed for both the frontal and the temporal M2 branches

tial anastomosis (Fig. 4.6). Linear arteriotomy was performed for both the frontal and the temporal M2 branches (Fig. 4.7). The lumina were flushed with heparinized saline, and the intima edges were marked with methylene blue.

The first anchor suture was placed, and knots were tied on the outside of the lumen. The tail of the suture thread was left in place (Fig. 4.8). On the other end of the stoma, a second anchor suture was placed, and knots were also tied in a similar

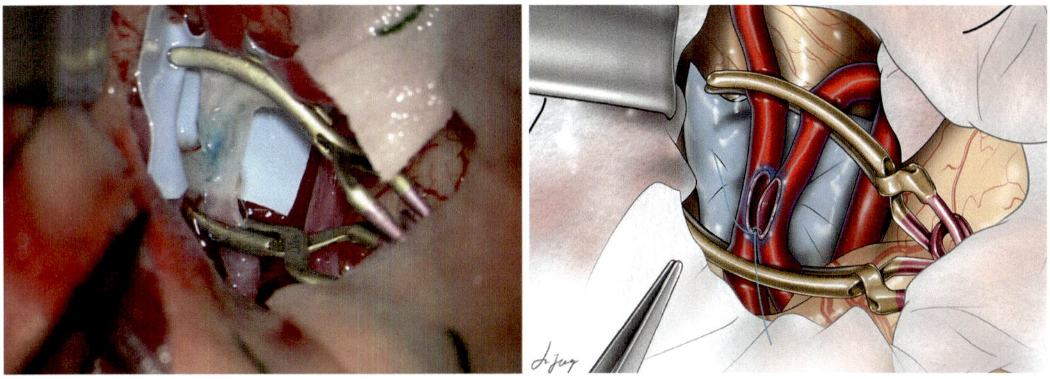

Fig. 4.8 The first anchor suture was placed, and knots were tied on the outside of the lumen. The tail of the suture thread was left in place

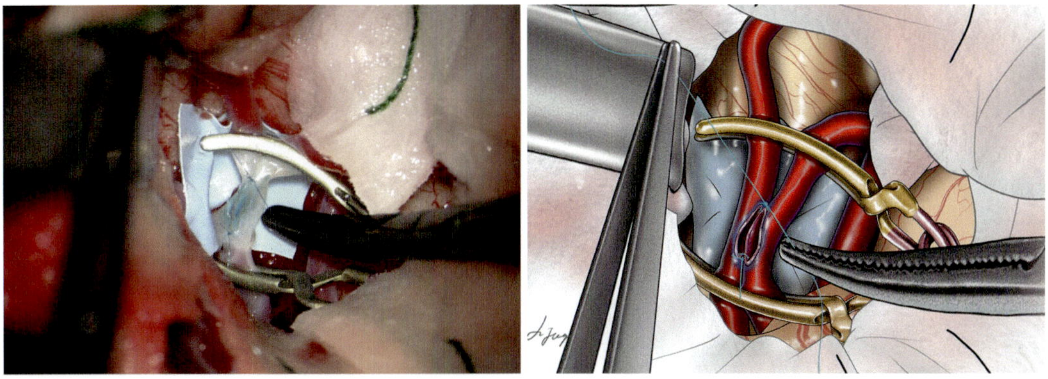

Fig. 4.9 A second anchor suture was placed, and knots were also tied in a similar fashion on the outside of the lumen

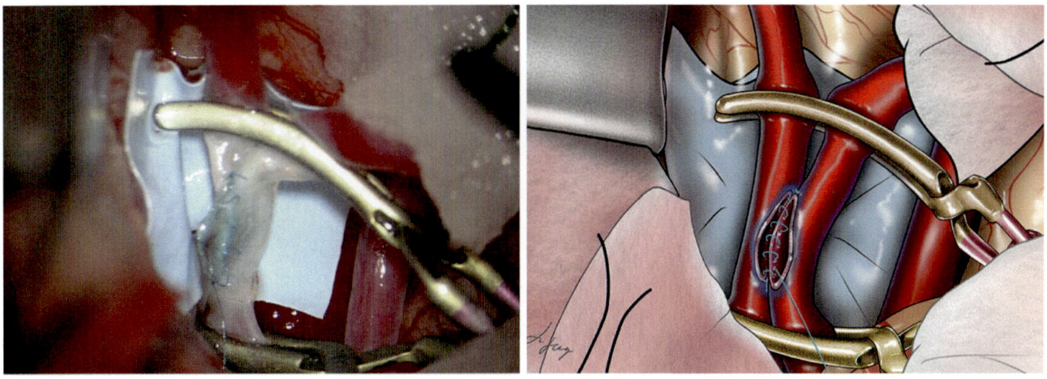

Fig. 4.10 Continuous suturing of the back wall was performed

fashion on the outside of the lumen (Fig. 4.9). Continuous suturing of the back wall was performed (Fig. 4.10), and the knot was tied with the suture thread left in place on the opposite anchor of the anastomosis (Fig. 4.11). Then, continuous suturing of the front wall was also performed (Fig. 4.12). Importantly, the intersuture distances were kept consistent. A second knot was tied with the suture thread left in place on the opposite anchor of the anastomosis (Fig. 4.13).

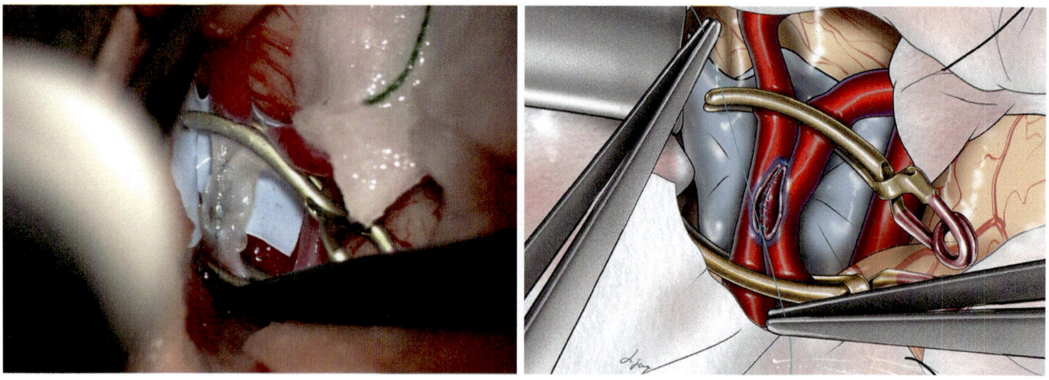

Fig. 4.11 The knot was tied with the suture thread left in place on the opposite anchor of the anastomosis

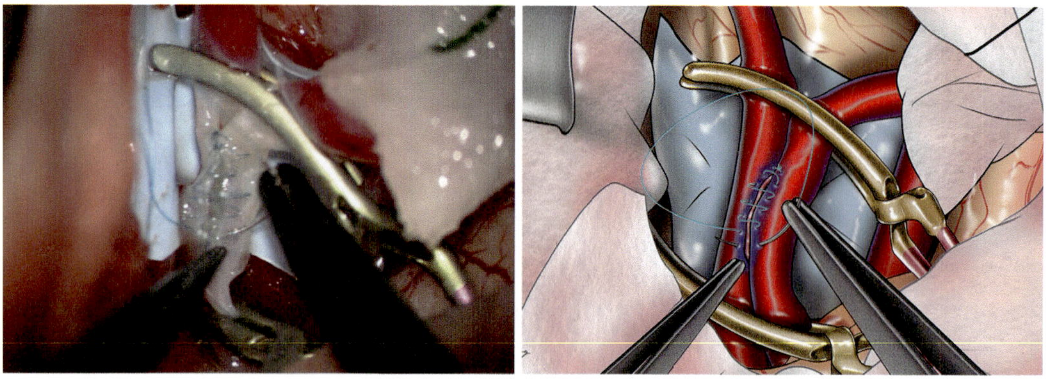

Fig. 4.12 Continuous suturing of the front wall was also performed

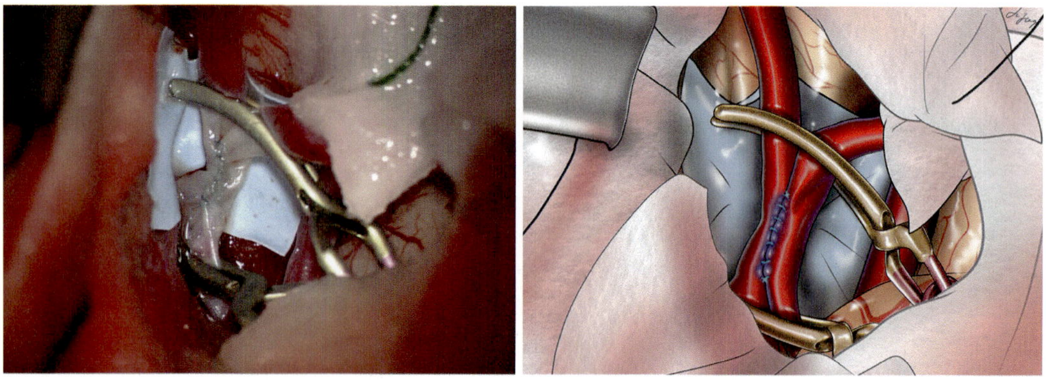

Fig. 4.13 The intersuture distances were kept consistent. A second knot was tied with the suture thread left in place on the opposite anchor of the anastomosis

Upon completion of the anastomosis, the temporary clips were removed, and a Doppler ultrasound probe was utilized to evaluate the anastomosis patency and flow status (Fig. 4.14). Small amounts of oozing could be stopped using Surgicel. The aneurysm was clipped distally and proximally, but the perforating artery was spared (Fig. 4.15).

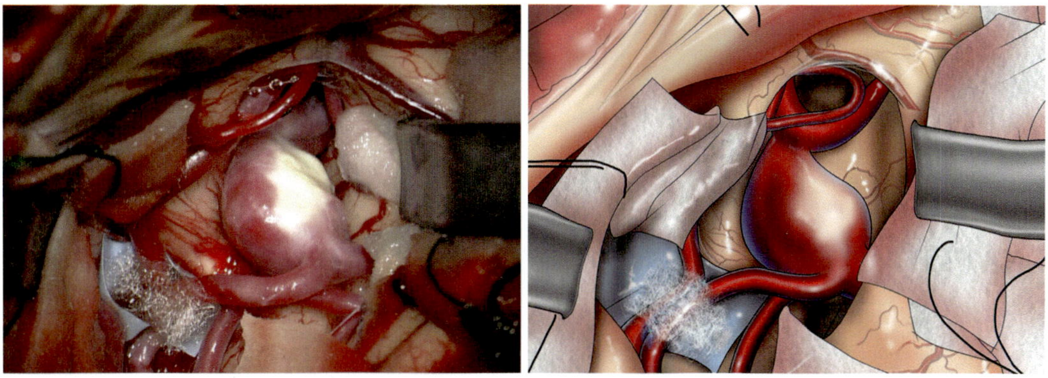

Fig. 4.14 Upon completion of the anastomosis, the temporary clips were removed, and a Doppler ultrasound probe was utilized to evaluate the anastomosis patency and flow status

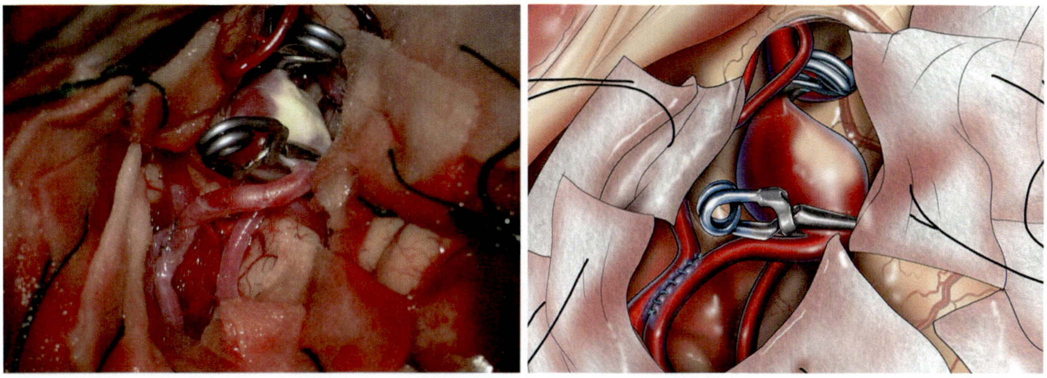

Fig. 4.15 The aneurysm was clipped distally and proximally, but the perforating artery was spared

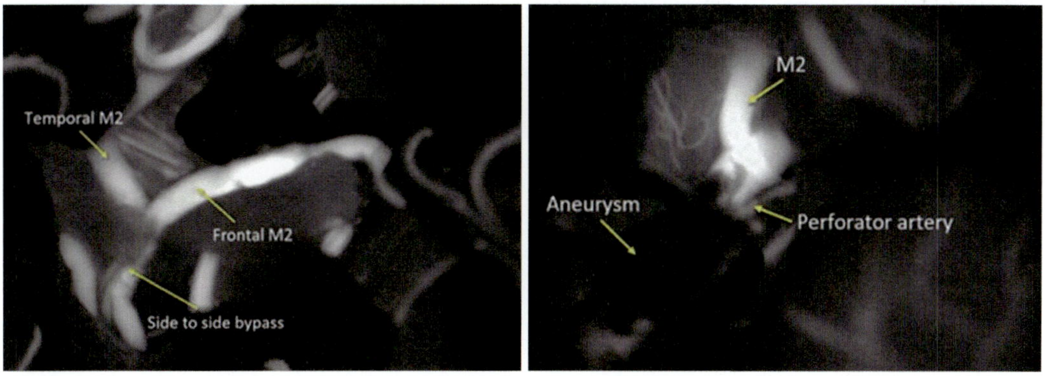

Fig. 4.16 Intraoperative indocyanine green angiography confirmed the patency of side-to-side bypass and satisfactory filling of the distal MCA, and the aneurysm was not visualized and had no blood supply

Intraoperative indocyanine green angiography and Doppler ultrasound confirmed the patency of side-to-side bypass and satisfactory filling of the distal MCA, and the aneurysm was not visualized and had no blood supply (Fig. 4.16). Postoperative DSA also showed patency of the anastomosis and obliteration of the aneurysm (Fig. 4.17).

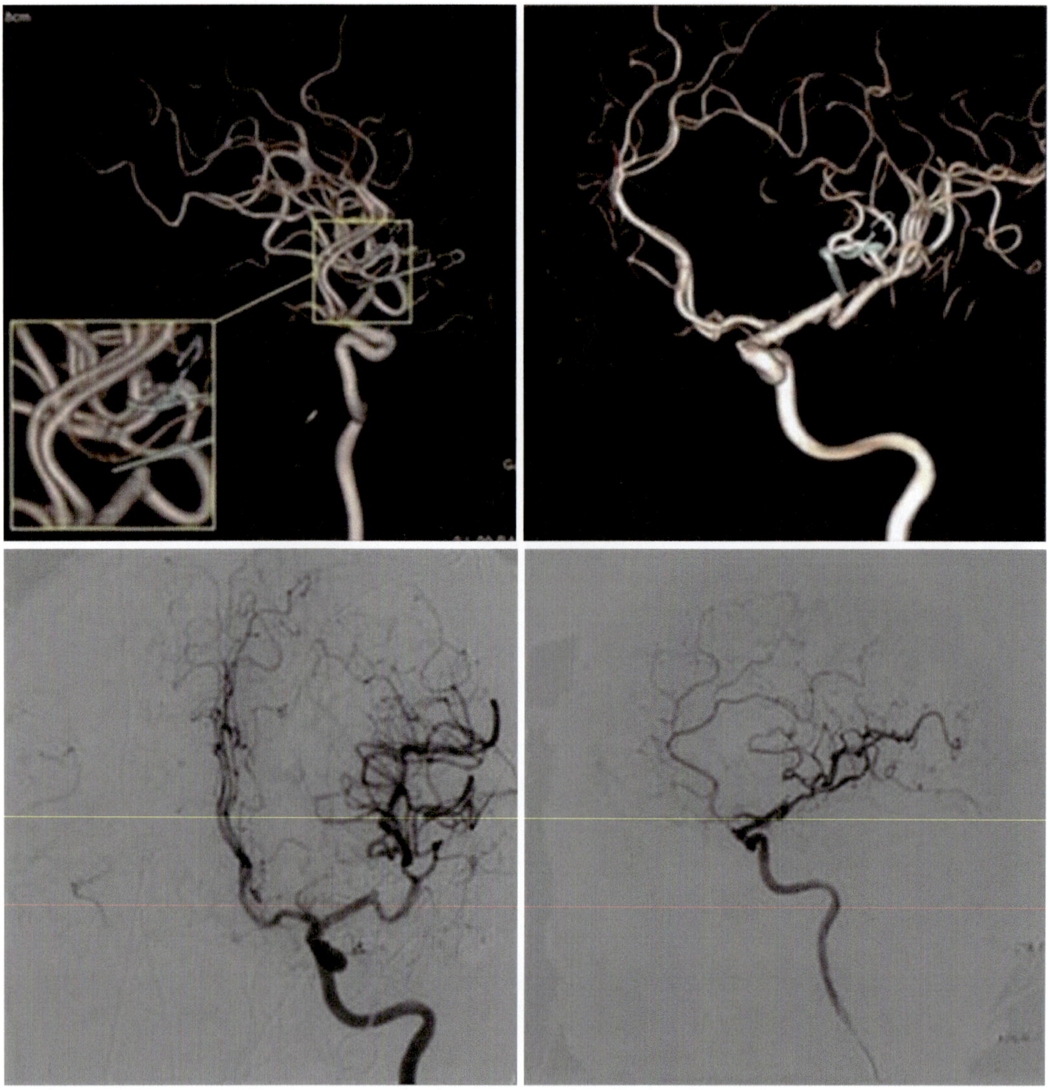

Fig. 4.17 Postoperative DSA also showed patency of the anastomosis and obliteration of the aneurysm

4.4 Comment

As described in Chapter 2, MCA-MCA (including M2-M2 or M3-M3) bypass is suitable for type B (aneurysms originating from the M2 segment or MCA bifurcation) and type C (aneurysms originating from the M3 or distal segments) MCA aneurysms [1]. Although it is challenging to perform side-to-side MCA-MCA anastomosis because of the limited mobility between arteries [2], we believe that this technique is somehow easier than end-to-side bypass. In our experience, widely opening the sylvian fissure and then holding both sides with a low-profile spatula can clearly expose the MCA vasculature, enabling dissection. Rapid revascularization should be considered to avoid ischemia when both MCA branches are temporarily occluded. However, due to the preferable matching and linear arteriotomy of both MCA branches, continuous suturing can quite smoothly and relatively easily performed. Additionally, there is no need to worry about the direction and length of the donor arteries, unlike during end-to-side EC-IC bypass. After the anastomosis was successfully completed, the relatively wide anastomotic stoma guarantees a high patency rate.

In addition, the anterior temporal artery (ATA), which is a proximal branch of the MCA, supplies nonsignificant regions of the brain and has a similar diameter to the secondary trunks of the MCA, is considered a promising donor source for side-to-side bypass of the MCA territory when feasible [3]. However, unlike distal MCA-MCA bypass, ATA-MCA bypass is always performed when M1 occlusion is required at the distal site of the ATA and has a higher risk of ischemia due to the requirement for temporary occlusion [4].

References

1. Zhu W, Liu P, Tian Y, Gu Y, Xu B, Chen L, Zhou L, Mao Y. Complex middle cerebral artery aneurysms: a new classification based on the angioarchitecture and surgical strategies. Acta Neurochir. 2013;155(8):1481–91.
2. Quinones-Hinojosa A, Lawton MT. In situ bypass in the management of complex intracranial aneurysms: technique application in 13 patients. Neurosurgery. 2005;57(1 Suppl):140–5. 140–45
3. Bederson JB, Spetzler RF. Anastomosis of the anterior temporal artery to a secondary trunk of the middle cerebral artery for treatment of a giant M1 segment aneurysm. Case report. J Neurosurg. 1992;76(5):863–6.
4. Sekhar LN, Natarajan SK, Britz GW, Ghodke B. Microsurgical management of anterior communicating artery aneurysms. Neurosurgery. 2007;61(5 Suppl 2):273–90.

5 Occipital Artery-Posterior Inferior Cerebellar Artery Bypass

Jianping Song and Wei Zhu

Abstract

Occipital artery (OA)-posterior inferior cerebellar artery (PICA) anastomosis was introduced as a crucial cerebral revascularization technique for the posterior circulation in the 1970s. The most suitable indications for OA-PICA bypass are complex and giant intracranial aneurysms involving the major vessels of the posterior circulation that cannot be secured by simple clipping or coiling. Additionally, the OA could also be used as a potential vessel source for bypass to treat vertebrobasilar insufficiency.

Keywords

Extracranial-intracranial bypass · Intracranial aneurysm · In situ bypass · Occipital artery Posterior inferior cerebellar artery Revascularization

5.1 Introduction

Occipital artery (OA)-posterior inferior cerebellar artery (PICA) anastomosis was introduced as a crucial cerebral revascularization technique for the posterior circulation in the 1970s [1–4]. The most suitable indications for OA-PICA bypass are complex and giant intracranial aneurysms involving the major vessels of the posterior circulation that cannot be secured by simple clipping or coiling. Additionally, the OA could also be used as a potential vessel source for bypass to treat vertebrobasilar insufficiency.

5.2 Case

A 68-year-old woman suffered from dizziness. Physical examination did not reveal any neurological deficits. Preoperative head computed tomography angiography (CTA) showed an aneurysm located at the vertebral artery (VA)-PICA junction. Enhanced high-resolution vessel wall magnetic resonance imaging (MRI) demonstrated focal enhancement of the aneurysmal wall (Fig. 5.1). Preoperative digital subtraction angiography (DSA) confirmed a left VA-PICA aneurysm, and the PICA originated from the aneurysmal wall (Fig. 5.2).

Endovascular treatment and direct clipping were not applicable. Therefore, to secure the aneurysm, left OA-PICA bypass combined with aneurysm trapping was planned for this patient (Fig. 5.3).

J. Song · W. Zhu (✉)
Huashan Hospital, Shanghai Medical College, Fudan University, Shanghai, China
e-mail: drzhuwei@fudan.edu.cn

Y. Mao et al. (eds.), *Surgical Atlas of Cerebral Revascularization*,
https://doi.org/10.1007/978-981-16-0374-7_5

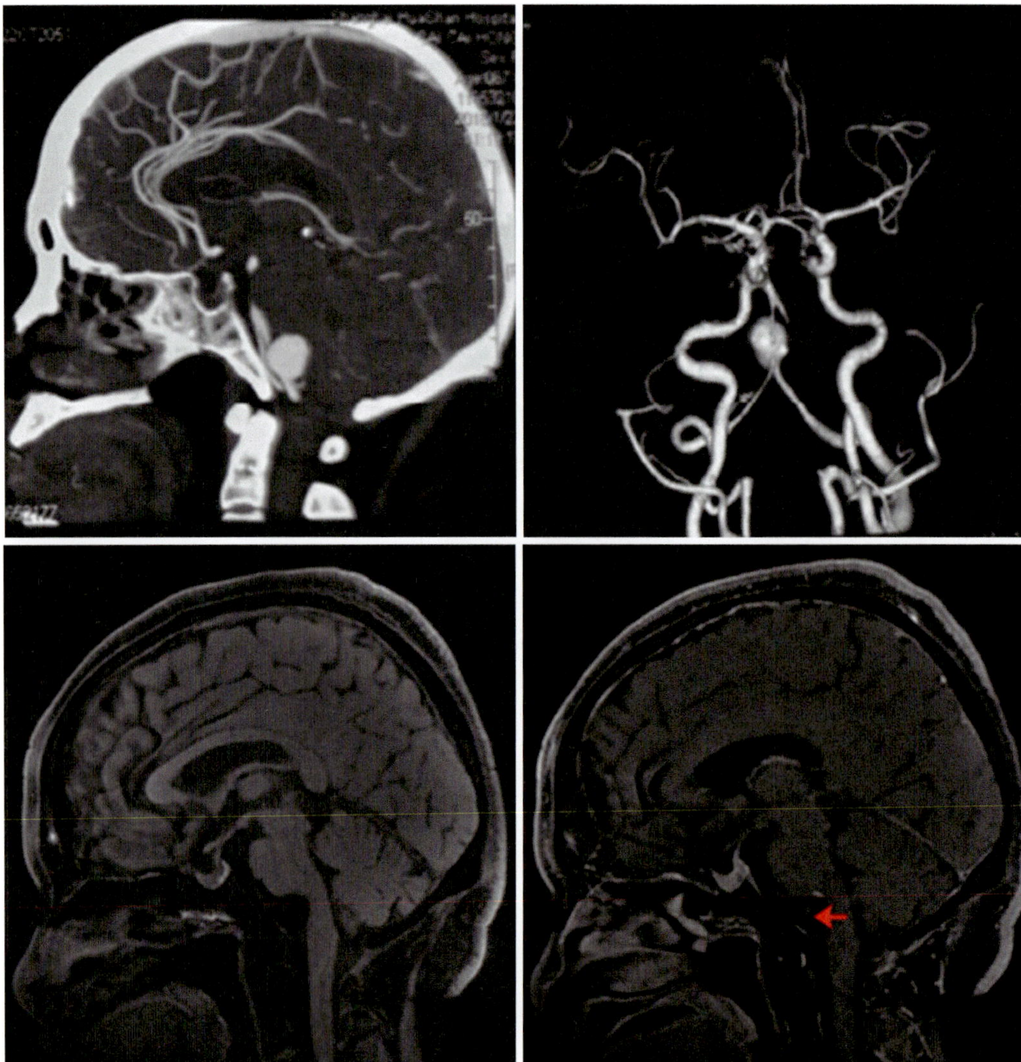

Fig. 5.1 Head CTA showed an aneurysm located at the VA-PICA junction. Enhanced high-resolution vessel wall MRI demonstrated focal enhancement of the aneurysmal wall (arrow)

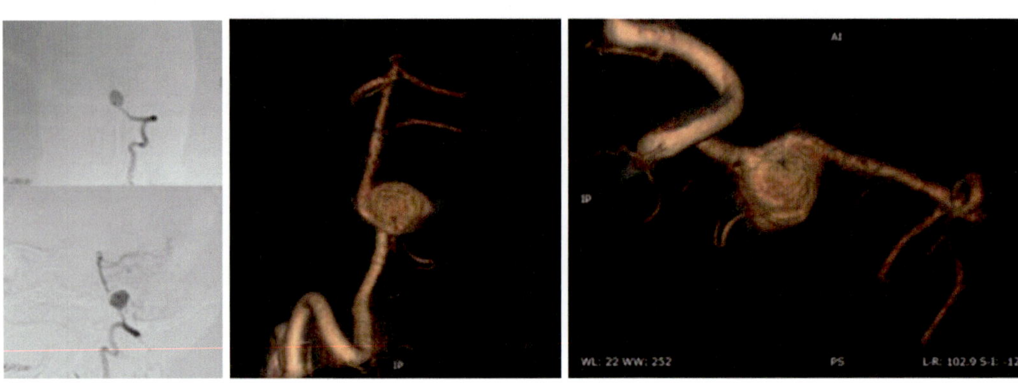

Fig. 5.2 Preoperative DSA confirmed a left VA-PICA aneurysm, and the PICA originated from the aneurysmal wall

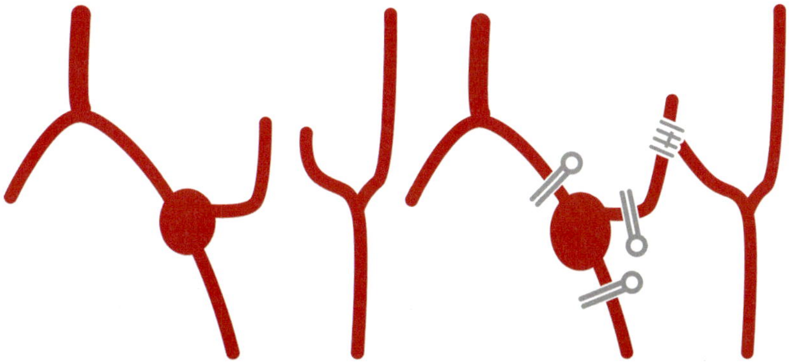

Fig. 5.3 Surgical plan: left OA-PICA bypass combined with aneurysm trapping

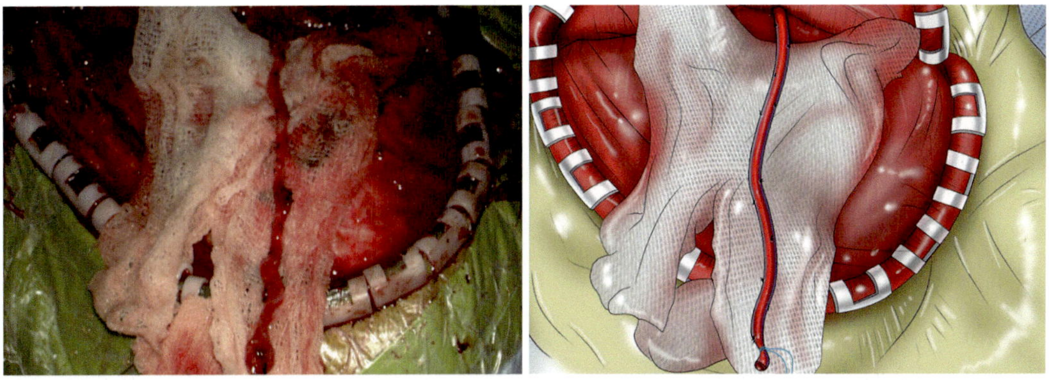

Fig. 5.4 The OA was skeletonized from the muscular skin flap in preparation for OA-PICA bypass

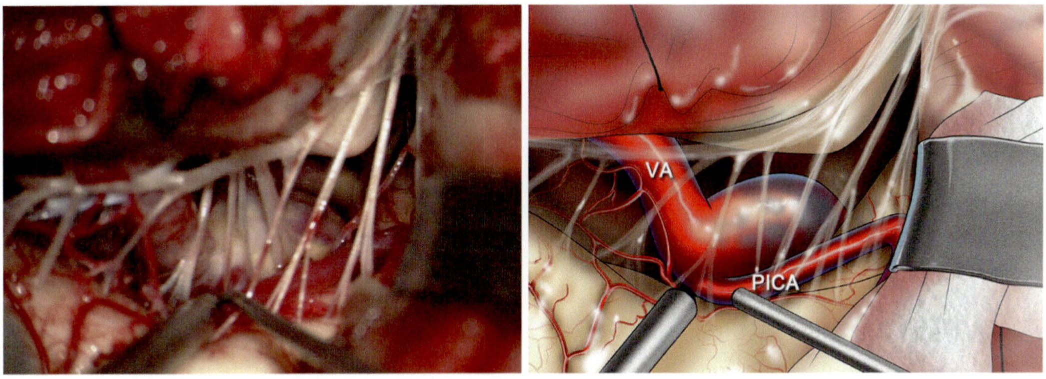

Fig. 5.5 The calcified aneurysm, the VA, and the anterior medullary segment of the PICA were exposed

5.3 Details of the Procedure

During the operation, the patient was placed in a park-bench position. We preferred the far-lateral approach with an inverted-L shape incision for craniotomy. The OA was skeletonized from the muscular skin flap in preparation for OA-PICA bypass (Fig. 5.4).

After performing craniotomy and opening the dura, the calcified aneurysm, the VA, and the anterior medullary segment of the PICA were exposed (Fig. 5.5). The lateral medullary and tonsillomedullary segments of the PICA were meticulously dissected from the adjacent tissues (Fig. 5.6). The tonsillomedullary segment of the PICA was determined as the recipient candidate for bypass. A rubber background was placed under the caudal loop of the tonsillomedullary segment of the PICA (Fig. 5.7).

The OA lumen was flushed with heparinized saline, and the intima edge was marked with methylene blue (Fig. 5.8). Temporary clips were

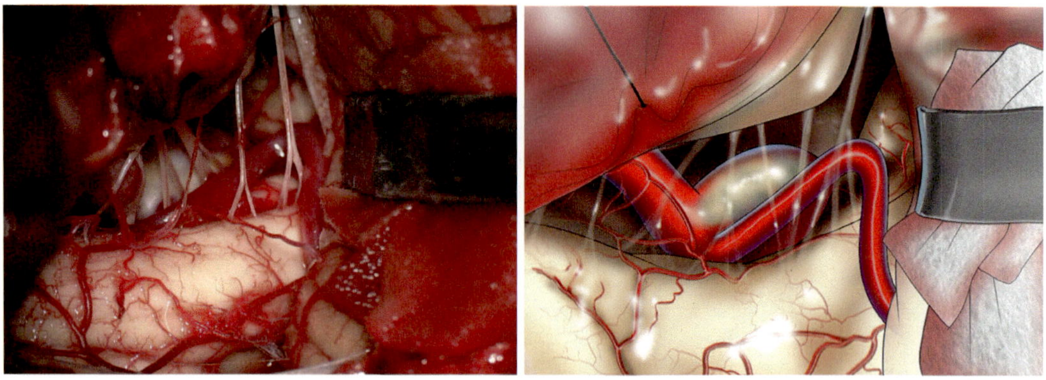

Fig. 5.6 The lateral medullary and tonsillomedullary segments of the PICA were meticulously dissected from the adjacent tissues

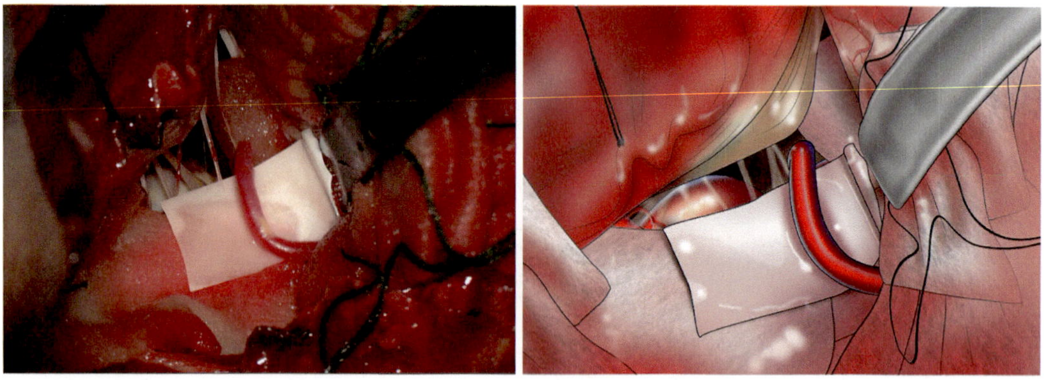

Fig. 5.7 The tonsillomedullary segment of the PICA was determined as the recipient candidate for bypass. A rubber background was placed under the caudal loop of the tonsillomedullary segment of the PICA

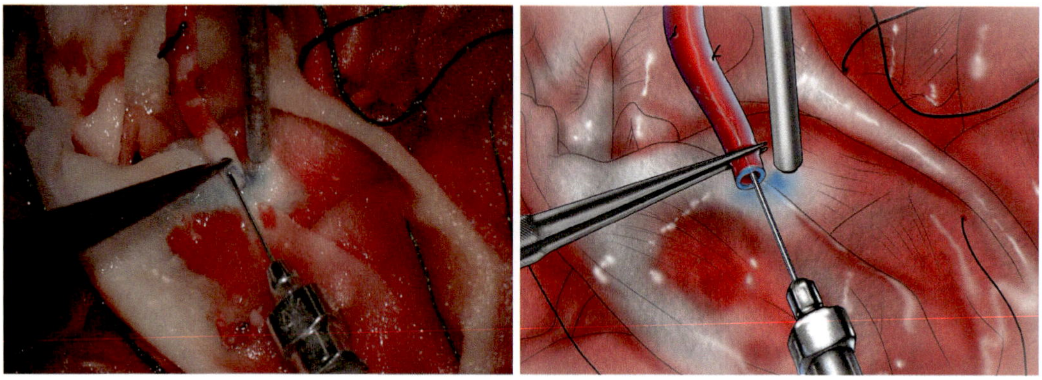

Fig. 5.8 The OA lumen was flushed with heparinized saline, and the intima edge was marked with methylene blue

placed on the proximal and distal ends of the recipient artery (Fig. 5.9). A linear arteriotomy was performed on the recipient artery, and an end-to-side anastomosis was achieved. Opposite anchor stitches (180° apart along the vessel circumference) were placed at the edge of the anastomosis (Fig. 5.10). First, 6–8 interrupted sutures were placed in the back wall of the anastomosis (Fig. 5.11). Then, the anastomotic stoma was gently rotated to suture the front wall in a similar interrupted fashion with 6–8 sutures (Fig. 5.12). After the anastomosis was complete (Fig. 5.13),

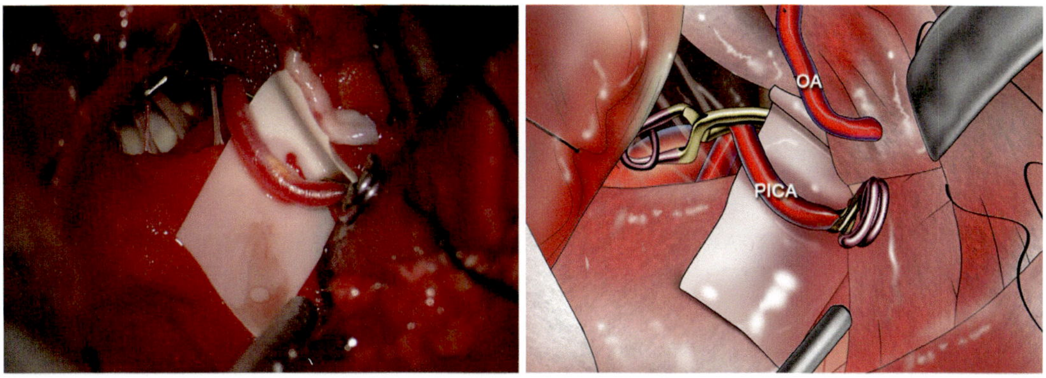

Fig. 5.9 Temporary clips were placed on the proximal and distal ends of the recipient artery

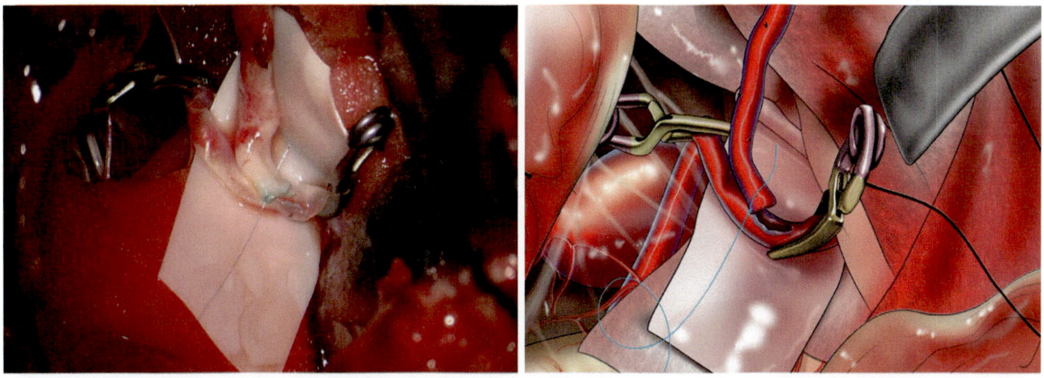

Fig. 5.10 An end-to-side anastomosis was achieved. Opposite anchor stitches (180° apart along the vessel circumference) were placed at the edge of the anastomosis

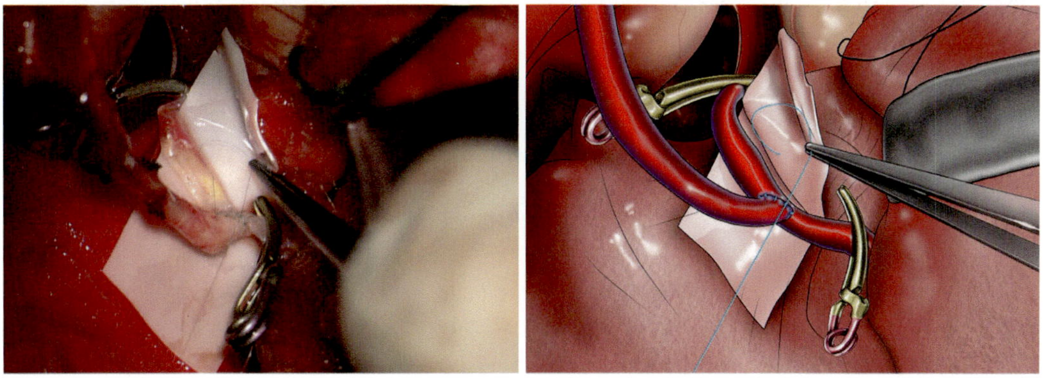

Fig. 5.11 First, 6–8 interrupted sutures were placed in the back wall of the anastomosis

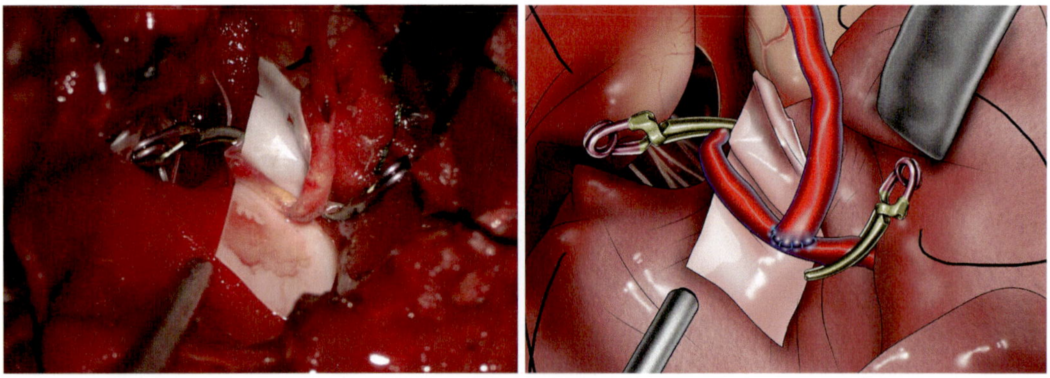

Fig. 5.12 The anastomotic stoma was gently rotated to suture the front wall in a similar interrupted fashion with 6–8 sutures

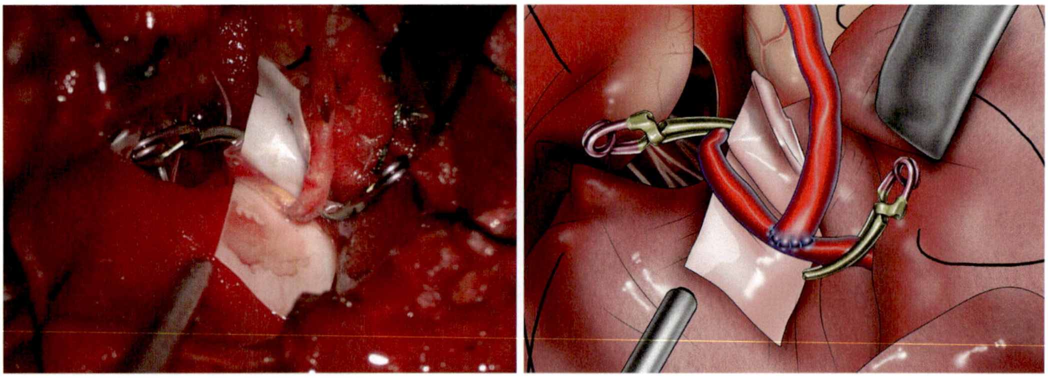

Fig. 5.13 The anastomosis was completed

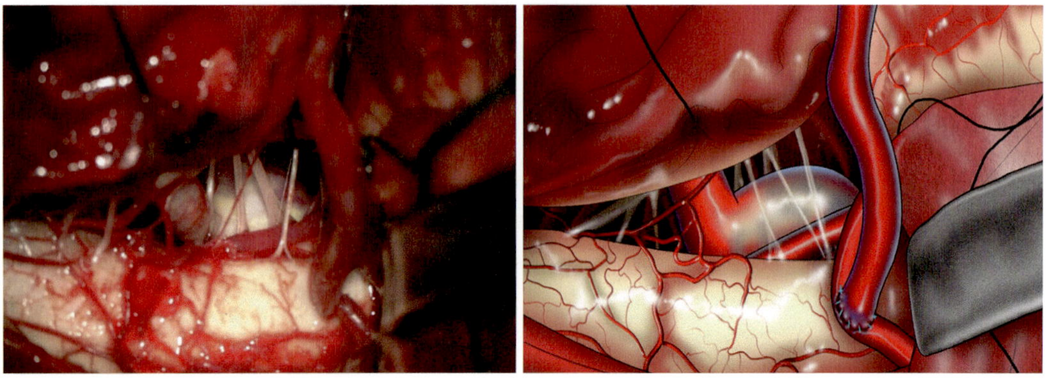

Fig. 5.14 The temporary clips on the OA were removed, and the patency of the anastomosis and the distal PICA were confirmed using a Doppler ultrasound probe

the temporary clips on the OA were removed, and the patency of the anastomosis and the distal PICA were confirmed using a Doppler ultrasound probe (Fig. 5.14). A small amount of oozing could be stopped using hemostasis materials.

Occlusion of the aneurysm was achieved by placing permanent clips on the VA proximal and distal to the aneurysm and the tosillomeduallry segment of the PICA proximal to the anastomosis (Fig. 5.15).

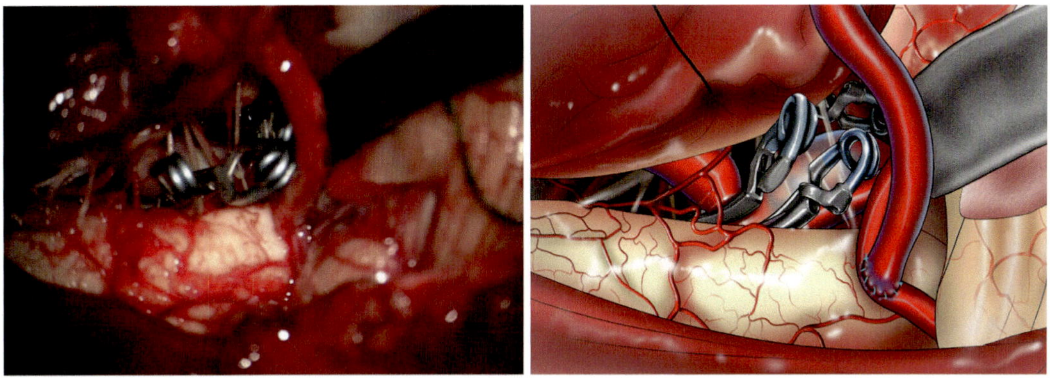

Fig. 5.15 Occlusion of the aneurysm was achieved by placing permanent clips on the VA proximal and distal to the aneurysm and the tonsillomedullary segment of the PICA proximal to the anastomosis

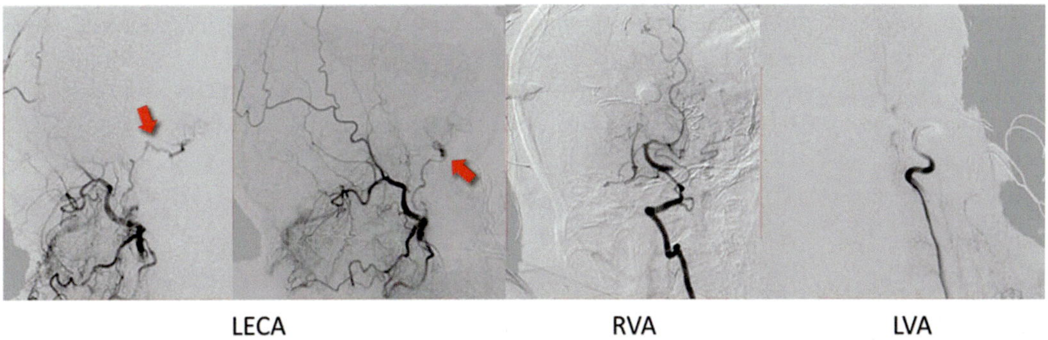

Fig. 5.16 Postoperative DSA showed patency of the OA-PICA bypass (arrow) and obliteration of the aneurysm

Postoperative DSA showed patency of the OA-PICA bypass (arrow) and obliteration of the aneurysm (Fig. 5.16).

5.4 Comment

Considering the OA's caliber, length, and flow volume, it could be an ideal donor for all posterior circulation distal branches revascularization [5, 6]. The OA originates from the external carotid artery and travels consistently through the inframastoid region [6, 7]. Then it curves upward to averagely 5 cm above the superior nuchal line [6, 8]. The OA has only small variations in this course. The mean diameters of the OA are 1.9 mm, 1.4 mm, and >1 mm at the orifice of the digastric groove, junction with the superior nuchal line, and the endpoint of the bifurcation [6, 8].

Adequate dissection of the OA is necessary for successful OA-PICA bypass surgery. However, OA harvesting is a technically challenging procedure due to the vessel's deep location and tortuous course between suboccipital muscles, especially for young neurosurgeons.

We usually performed a far-lateral approach with an inverted L-shape incision. Typically, the upper horizontal incision line of the inverted "L" should be at least 2 cm higher than the superior nuchal line to obtain a sufficient length of OA for bypass surgery. At the superior nuchal line, the OA is about is 2.5 cm lateral to the external occipital protuberance in women and 4 cm in men, and can be located with ultrasound or simple palpation [6, 9].

Based on the literature and the authors' experience, there are two popular kinds of OA harvesting techniques in clinical practice, and we describe them as follows:

The first and classic technique of OA harvesting is the retrograde technique (from the distal end to the proximal end); this is usually performed in a "layer-by-layer" fashion, which means dissecting the OA from the surrounding muscles according to its anatomic relations. The subcutaneous segment is detected by palpation or Doppler ultrasound and outlined with a skin marker. We use a microscope to perform OA dissection after the initial superficial incision was performed, and the skin flap was mobilized. We firstly dissect the subcutaneous segment from the epigaleal layer and the transitional segment from multiple muscle layers. Then we harvest the intramuscular segment down to the mastoid groove. It is important to leave a periadventitial cuff along the OA to prevent spasm. Usually, there will be a large muscular branch originated from the OA proximally. The muscular branch should be carefully identified, coagulated, and transected. The OA should be dissected proximally until its entrance into the muscular bed at the mastoid groove, and the dissection can be continued after removal of the styloid diaphragm until the posterior margin of the longissimus capitis muscle [10]. We advocate a total length of 10–15 cm of OA to be freed. The maneuver ensures the OA can reach the anastomosis site with extra length and further avoid any sutures' tension [10, 11].

The second OA harvesting technique is anterograde dissection (from the proximal end to the distal end). This technique was first described by Sundt TJ et al. [12] and further developed and renamed the transperiosteal "inside-out" technique by Lawton MT et al. [13]. We also had a similar idea and conducted OA harvesting using anterograde dissection in recent years (Fig. 5.17).

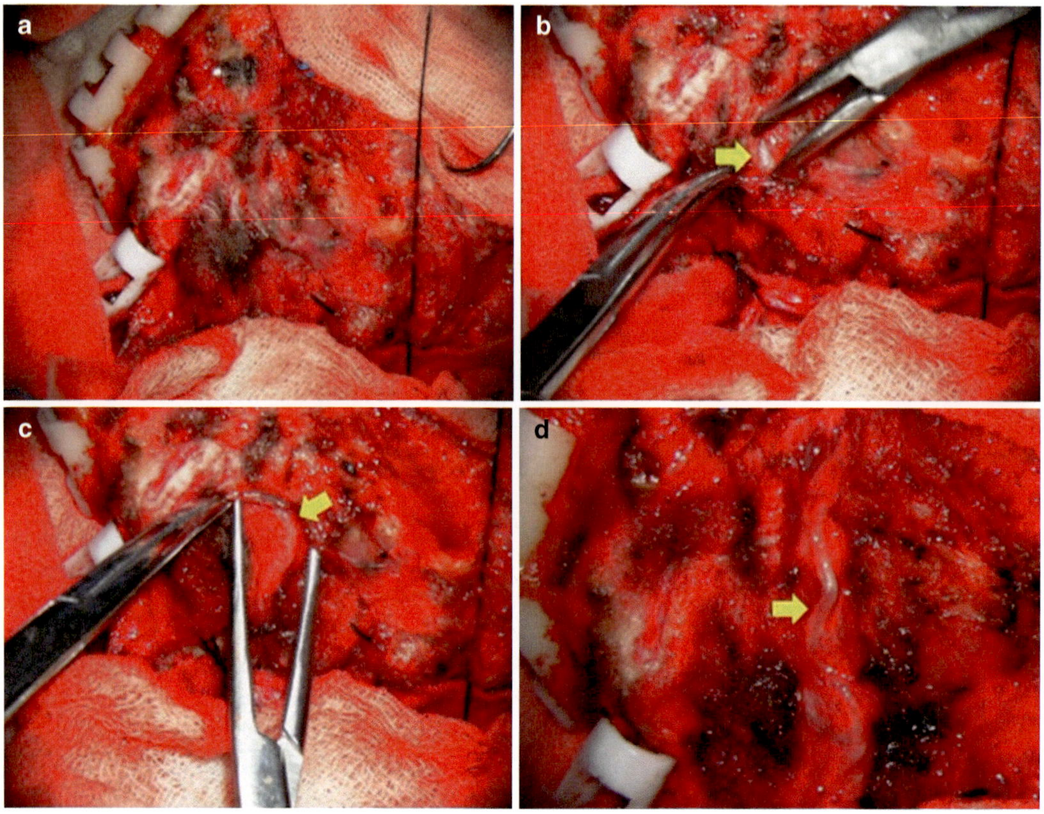

Fig. 5.17 After the one-piece myocutaneous flap is established (**a**), the OA can be identified by palpation or Doppler ultrasound. The intramuscular space was opened by blunt dissection to localize the OA (arrow) (**b**). The dissection can be continuously performed (**c**), and the OA was freed in a proximal to distal direction (**d**)

The major difference between the retrograde and anterograde techniques is that the latter usually uses a one-piece myocutaneous flap instead of a skin flap. The myocutaneous flap, including the nuchal muscles and the OA's distal part, is carefully mobilized after the incision. The digastric muscle and its groove, the occipital groove, and the superior oblique muscle are key landmarks to identify the OA's intramuscular segment. This approach also avoids critical neurovascular structures impingement such as the VA. A transperiosteal "inside-out" approach is then used to harvest the OA, by identifying the vessel at the occipital groove and freeing it through the periosteum [14]. The OA is then harvested anterogradely until the skin incision was reached within the flap.

In our opinion, the basic goal of these two techniques is to expose the easiest part of OA first and then dissect the vessel along the rest of the artery. The retrograde technique needs a thorough understanding of the anatomy due to the "layer-to-layer" dissection; in contrast, the anterograde technique only needs a single one-piece myocutaneous flap, which is easier for young neurosurgeons to establish. However, the risk of OA injury during myocutaneous flap mobilization may be higher than that during "layer-to-layer" dissection if the dissection is not strictly maintained under the periosteum. The OA's subcutaneous and intramuscular segments are the easiest to identify with the retrograde and anterograde techniques, respectively. In both techniques, dissection of the OA's transitional segment is the most difficult to perform due to the tight tissue layers surrounding the artery. The bellies of the sternocleidomastoid muscle and the semispinalis muscle can be used as landmarks for localizing the OA's transitional segment. Currently, in our practice, we dissect the OA with a modified method. We now create a single myocutaneous flap and identify and free the subcutaneous and intramuscular segments of the OA first, and then the transitional segment of OA is finally dissected, assisted by Doppler ultrasound. Because both sides of the transitional segment have been exposed, the risk of dissecting this segment in the wrong direction can be minimized. We believe that this modified technique combines the benefits of both the abovementioned anterograde and retrograde techniques.

References

1. Spetzler R, Chater N. Occipital artery--middle cerebral artery anastomosis for cerebral artery occlusive disease. Surg Neurol. 1974;2(4):235–8.
2. Ausman JI, Lee MC, Klassen AC, Seljeskog EL, Chou SN. Stroke: what's new? Cerebral revascularization. Minn Med. 1976;59(4):223–7.
3. Khodadad G. Occipital artery-posterior inferior cerebellar artery anastomosis. Surg Neurol. 1976;5(4):225–7.
4. Sundt TJ, Whisnant JP, Piepgras DG, Campbell JK, Holman CB. Intracranial bypass grafts for vertebral-basilar ischemia. Mayo Clin Proc. 1978;53(1):12–8.
5. Ates O, Ahmed AS, Niemann D, Baskaya MK. The occipital artery for posterior circulation bypass: microsurgical anatomy. Neurosurg Focus. 2008;24(2):E9.
6. Mao Y. Revascularization with the occipital artery to treat aneurysms in the posterior circulation. World Neurosurg. 2014;82(3–4):e415–6.
7. Uchino A, Saito N, Mizukoshi W, Okada Y. Anomalous origin of the occipital artery diagnosed by magnetic resonance angiography. Neuroradiology. 2011;53(11):853–7.
8. Alvernia JE, Fraser K, Lanzino G. The occipital artery: a microanatomical study. Neurosurgery. 2006;58(1 Suppl):S114–22.
9. Arai T, Ishikawa K, Saito T, Hashimoto Y, Asai T, Okuda Y. Distance from the external occipital protuberance to the occipital artery for occipital nerve block. J Anesth. 2013;27(5):801–2.
10. Katsuno M, Tanikawa R, Uemori G, Kawasaki K, Izumi N, Hashimoto M. Occipital artery-to-posterior inferior cerebellar artery anastomosis with multiple-layer dissection of suboccipital muscles under a reverse C-shaped skin incision. Br J Neurosurg. 2015;29(3):401–5.
11. Nossek E, Chalif DJ, Dehdashti AR. How I do it: occipital artery to posterior inferior cerebellar artery bypass. Acta Neurochir. 2014;156(5):971–5.
12. Sundt TJ, Piepgras DG. Occipital to posterior inferior cerebellar artery bypass surgery. J Neurosurg. 1978;48(6):916–28.
13. Benet A, Tabani H, Ding X, Burkhardt J, Rodriguez Rubio R, Tayebi Meybodi A, Nisson P, Kola O, Gandhi S, Yousef S, Lawton MT. The transperiosteal "inside-out" occipital artery harvesting technique. J Neurosurg. 2018;130(1):207–12.
14. Tabani H, Gandhi S, Burkhardt JK, Benet A, Lawton MT. Transperisosteal "Inside out" occipital artery harvest and occipital artery-anterior inferior cerebellar artery bypass for vertebrobasilar ischemia: 3-dimensional operative video. Oper Neurosurg (Hagerstown); 2017.

Posterior Inferior Cerebellar Artery-Vertebral Artery Bypass

6

Kai Quan, Xin Zhang, and Wei Zhu

Abstract

Intracranial-intracranial (IC-IC) bypass could be a feasible option when the V4 is long enough and the posterior inferior cerebellar artery (PICA)-vertebral artery (VA) can be transected and reimplanted into the V4 using an end-to-side anastomosis technique. PICA-VA bypasses spare the neurosurgeon from the tedious dissection required to harvest the occipital artery (OA) or expose the extradural VA for extracranial-IC (EC-IC) bypass. The indications for PICA-VA reimplantation bypass are proximal complex PICA aneurysms, including the PICA-VA junction, P1, and P2 aneurysms.

Keywords

Intracranial aneurysm · Intracranial-intracranial bypass · Posterior inferior cerebellar artery · Reimplantation Revascularization bypass · Vertebral artery

6.1 Introduction

Intracranial-intracranial (IC-IC) bypass could be a feasible option when the V4 is long enough and the posterior inferior cerebellar artery (PICA)-vertebral artery (VA) can be transected and reimplanted into the V4 using an end-to-side anastomosis technique. PICA-VA bypasses spare the neurosurgeon from the tedious dissection required to harvest the occipital artery (OA) or expose the extradural VA for extracranial-IC (EC-IC) bypass [1]. The indications for PICA-VA reimplantation bypass are proximal complex PICA aneurysms, including the PICA-VA junction, P1, and P2 aneurysms.

6.2 Case

A 60-year-old woman suffered from sudden-onset unconsciousness after drinking 5 days prior. Physical examination before the operation showed that her Glasgow coma score was 13, with a positive Kernig sign. The preoperative head computed tomography (CT) showed subarachnoid and fourth ventricle hemorrhage (Fig. 6.1). Digital subtraction angiography (DSA) confirmed a right PICA dissecting aneurysm (Fig. 6.2).

Endovascular treatment and direct clipping were not applicable. Therefore, considering the high originating location of the PICA, a PICA-VA reimplantation bypass combined with aneurysm trapping was planned for this patient (Fig. 6.3).

K. Quan · X. Zhang · W. Zhu (✉)
Huashan Hospital, Shanghai Medical College, Fudan University, Shanghai, China
e-mail: drzhuwei@fudan.edu.cn

Y. Mao et al. (eds.), *Surgical Atlas of Cerebral Revascularization*,
https://doi.org/10.1007/978-981-16-0374-7_6

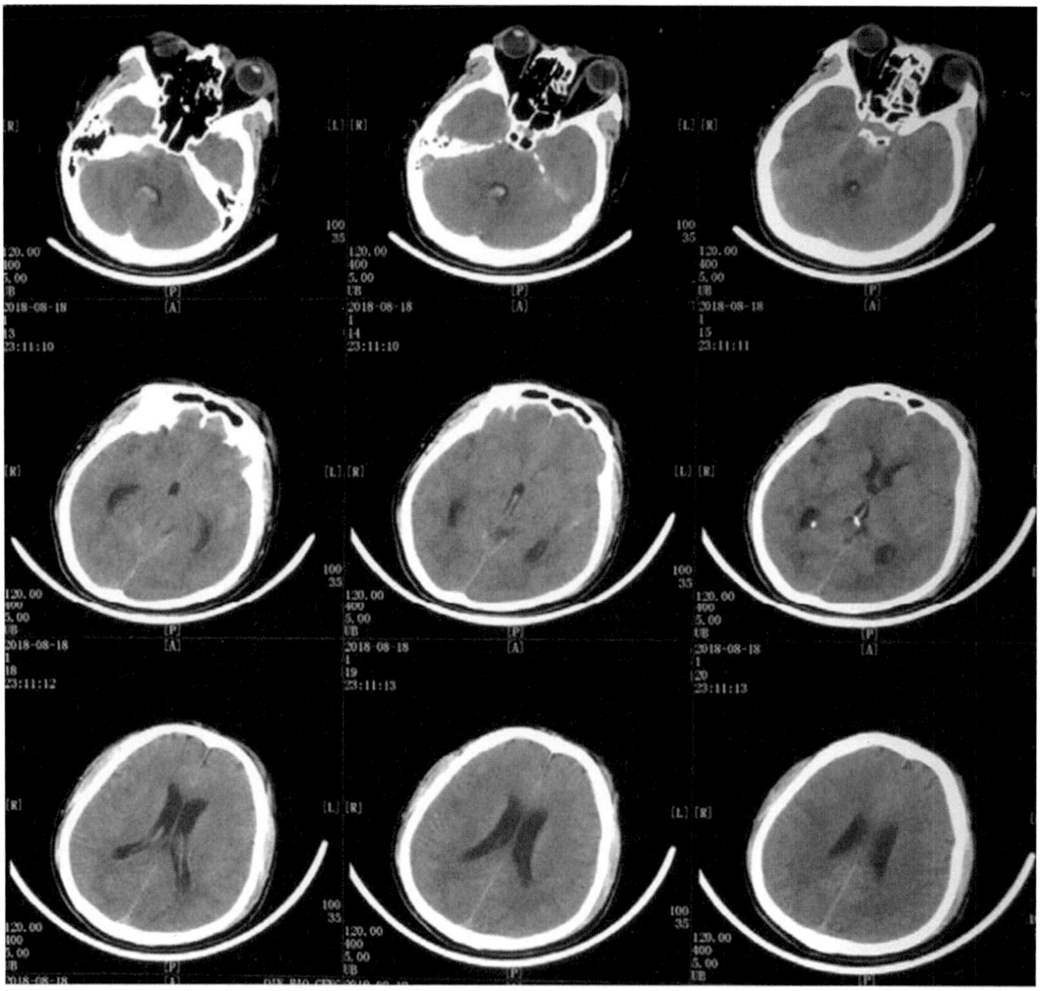

Fig. 6.1 The preoperative head CT showed subarachnoid and fourth ventricle hemorrhage

6.3 Details of the Procedure

During the operation, the patient was placed in a left park-bench position, and a right far-lateral approach was applied. After performing craniotomy and opening the dura, the right VA and PICA were exposed carefully under the microscope. Due to the high originating location of the PICA, a sufficient length of the VA V3 segment could be used for reimplantation bypass. A temporary clip was placed at the proximal segment of the VA to obtain proximal control of PICA inflow to prevent premature rupture of the aneurysm during dissection (Fig. 6.4).

Then, the aneurysm was inspected. The aneurysm was located at the PICA P1/P2 segment and was obviously larger than what we observed on DSA. During dissection of the PICA, a hematoma was observed around the aneurysm. (Fig. 6.5). The PICA proximal to the aneurysm was dissected, exposed carefully (Fig. 6.6), and then clipped (Fig. 6.7).

A segment of the intradural VA (V3) was temporarily clipped with two clips, setting the reimplantation site (Fig. 6.8). As the recipient artery, the PICA loop distal to the aneurysm was clipped and was intended for reimplantation in the intradural VA (Fig. 6.9). The PICA distal to the aneu-

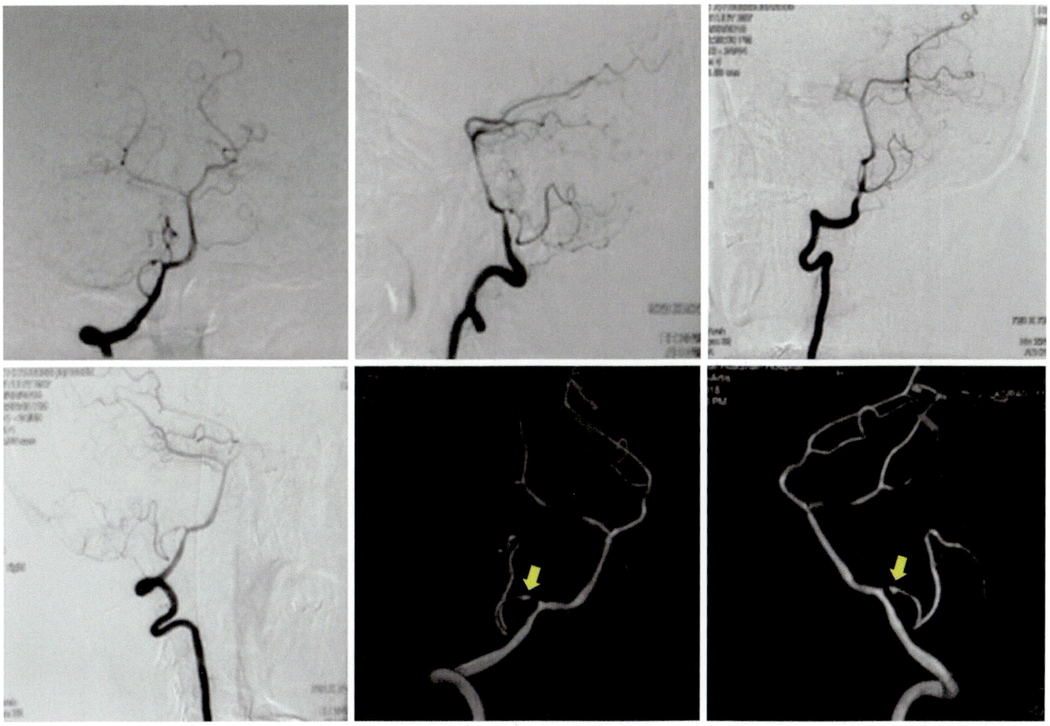

Fig. 6.2 Preoperative DSA confirmed a right PICA dissecting aneurysm

Fig. 6.3 Surgical plan: right PICA-VA reimplantation bypass combined with aneurysm trapping

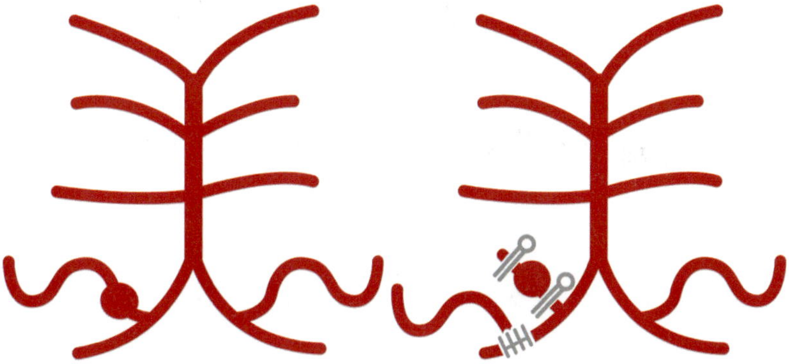

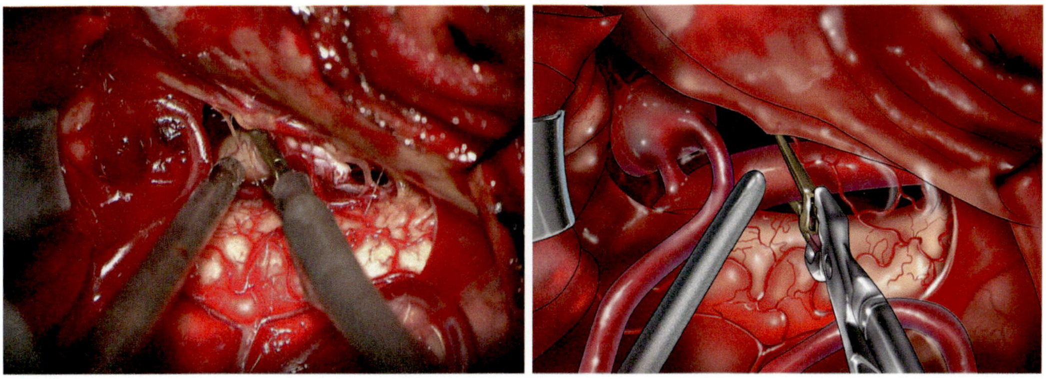

Fig. 6.4 Due to the high originating location of the PICA, a sufficient length of the VA V3 segment could be used for reimplantation bypass. A temporary clip was placed at the proximal segment of the VA

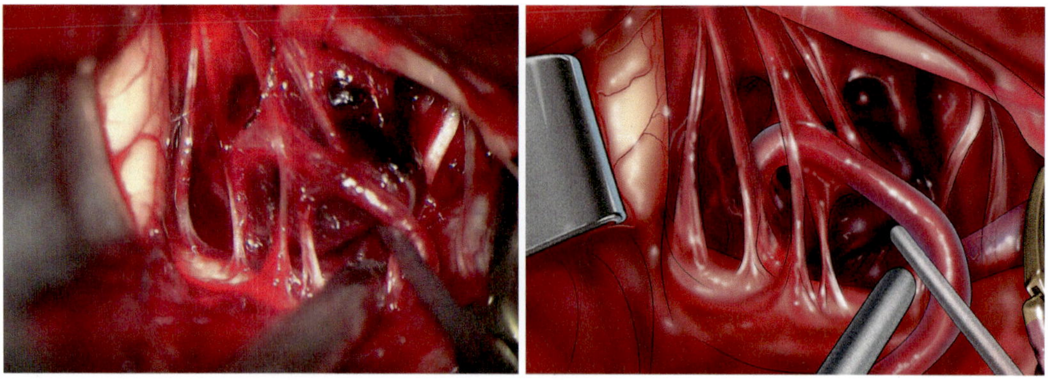

Fig. 6.5 During dissection of the PICA, a hematoma was observed around the aneurysm

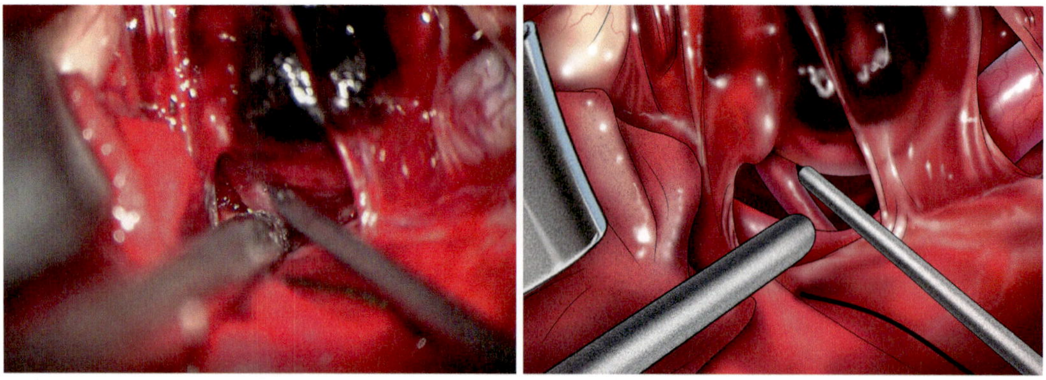

Fig. 6.6 The PICA proximal to the aneurysm was dissected and exposed carefully

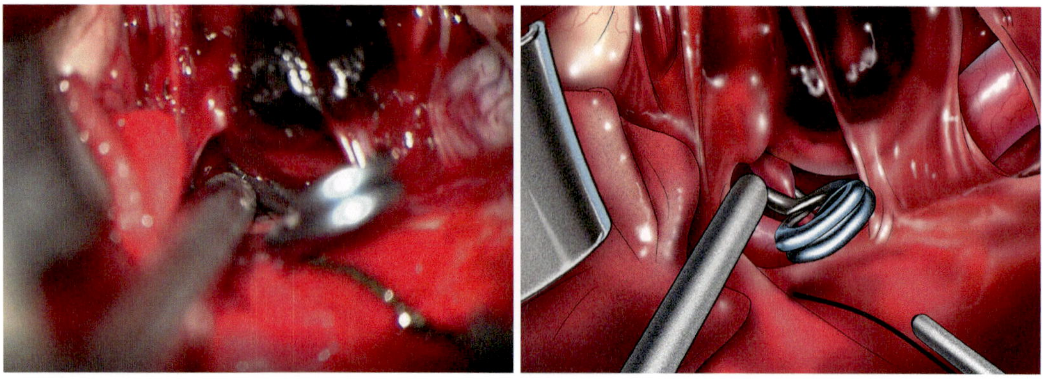

Fig. 6.7 The PICA was clipped proximally

rysm was cut, and the aneurysm was trapped. The edge of the lumen was marked by methylene blue. A cotton pad was placed to protect the medulla (Fig. 6.10). The reimplantation site on the intradural VA was cut in a fish-mouth fashion, and the artery lumina was flushed with heparinized saline (Fig. 6.11). An end-to-side anastomosis strategy was applied for PICA-VA suturing. The first anchor suture was placed at the distal corner of the anastomotic stoma (Fig. 6.12). An

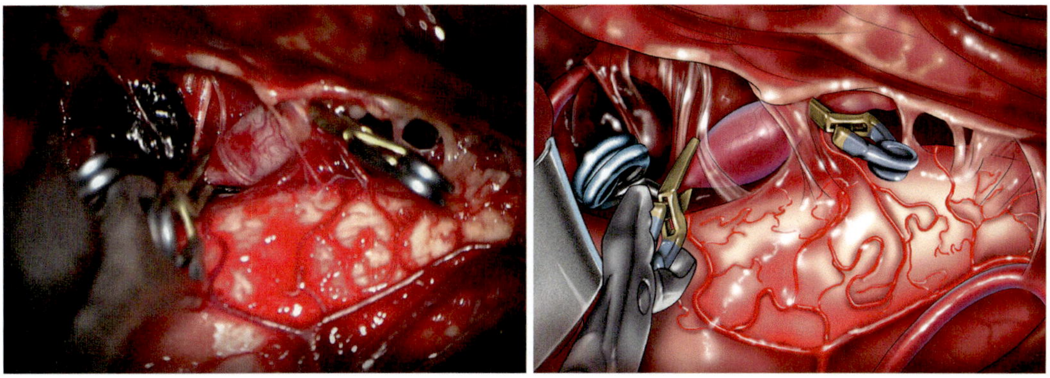

Fig. 6.8 A segment of the intradural VA (V3) was temporarily clipped with two clips, setting the reimplantation site

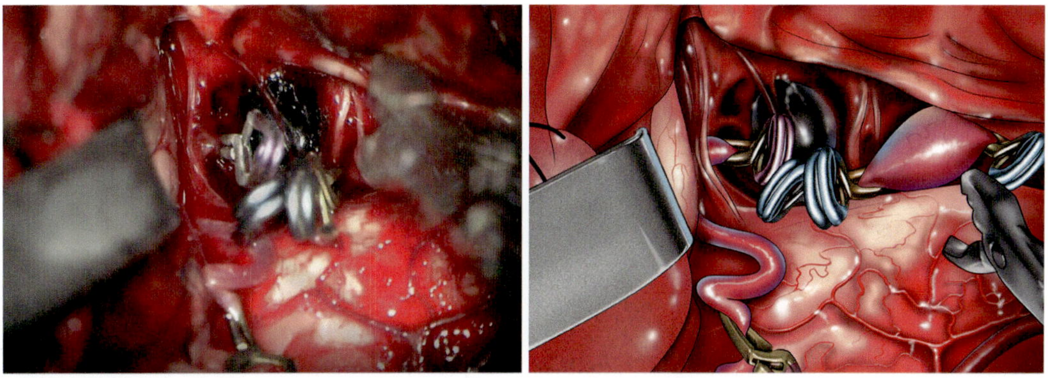

Fig. 6.9 As the recipient artery, the PICA loop distal to the aneurysm was clipped and was intended for reimplantation in the intradural VA

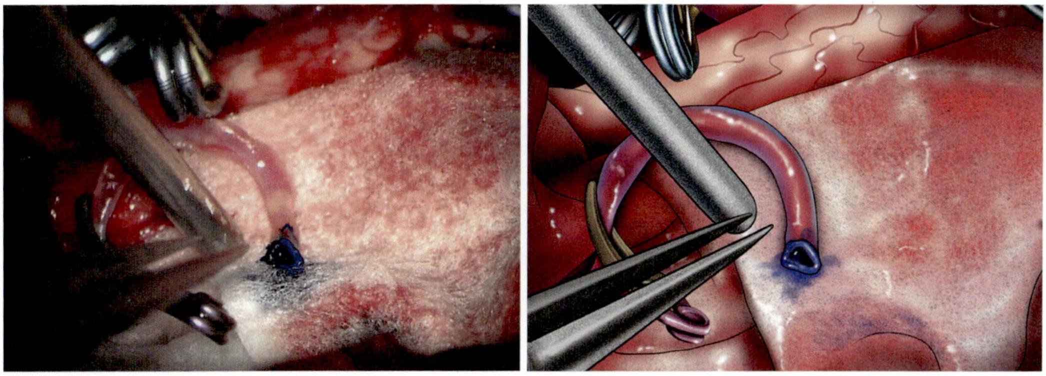

Fig. 6.10 The PICA distal to the aneurysm was cut, and the aneurysm was trapped. The edge of the lumen was marked by methylene blue. A cotton pad was placed to protect the medulla

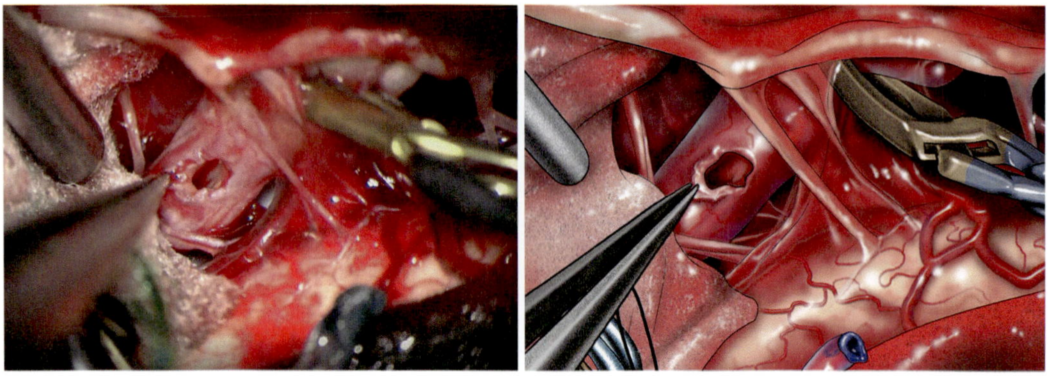

Fig. 6.11 The reimplantation site on the intradural VA was cut in a fish-mouth fashion, and the artery lumina was flushed with heparinized saline

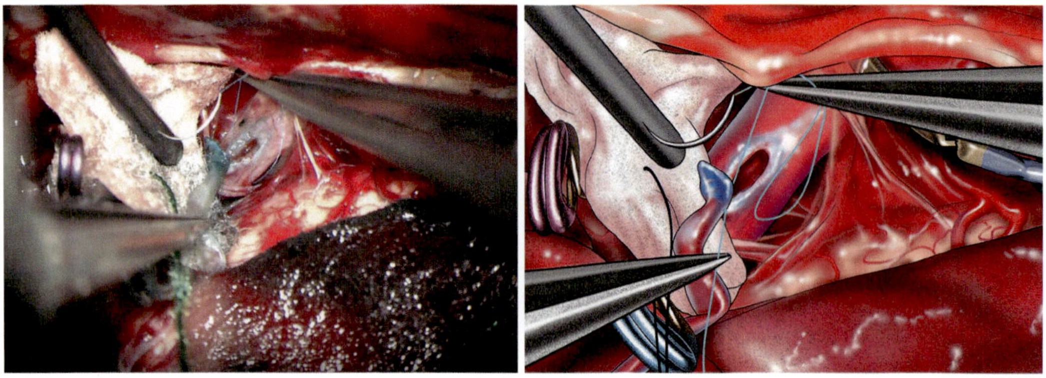

Fig. 6.12 An end-to-side anastomosis strategy was applied for PICA-VA suturing. The first anchor suture was placed at the distal corner of the anastomotic stoma

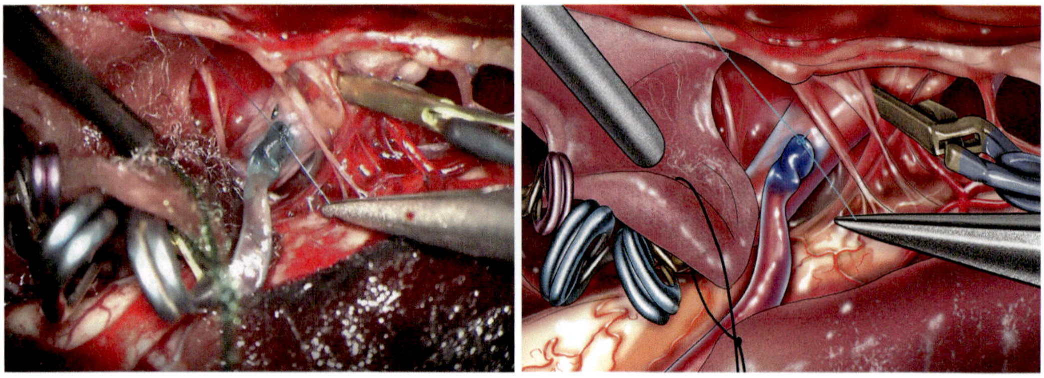

Fig. 6.13 An opposite anchor suture (180° apart along the vessel circumference) was placed at the other edge of the anastomosis

opposite anchor suture (180° apart along the vessel circumference) was placed at the other edge of the anastomosis (Fig. 6.13). Next, 6–8 interrupted sutures were placed in the front wall with intervals of 1–2 mm (Figs. 6.14 and 6.15). Then, the PICA was rotated gently, and the back wall of

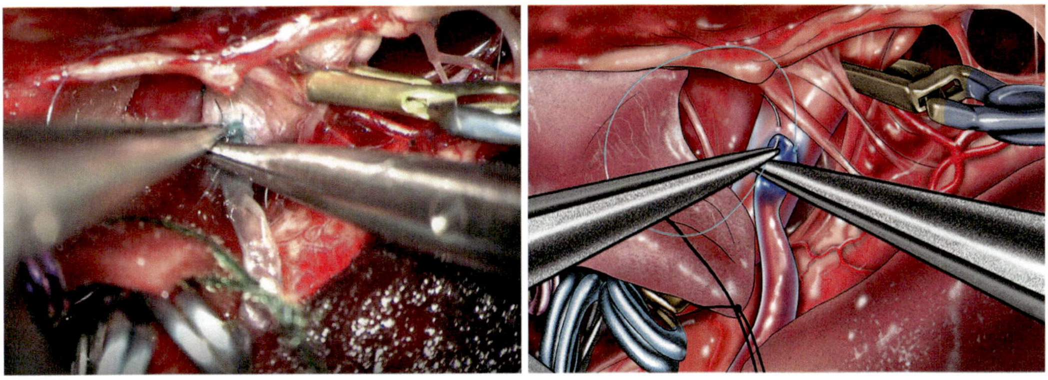

Fig. 6.14 Interrupted sutures were placed in the front wall with intervals of 1–2 mm

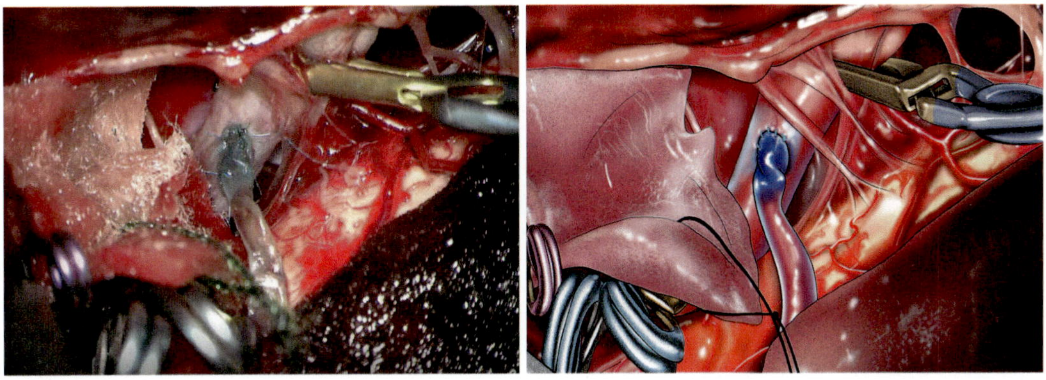

Fig. 6.15 The front wall was sutured with 6–8 stitches

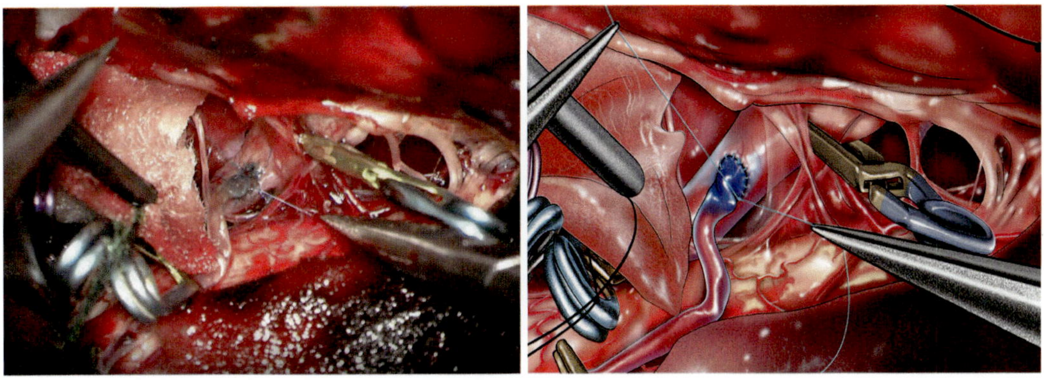

Fig. 6.16 The PICA was gently rotated; 6–8 interrupted sutures were also placed in the back wall of the stoma

the stoma was also sutured interruptedly with 6–8 stitches (Fig. 6.16). After bypass was completed, the temporary clips were removed to check for oozing from the anastomotic stoma, and additional stitches were placed to stop the bleeding, if necessary. A Doppler probe was used to confirm the patency of the PICA. Surgicel and bioglue were applied to reinforce the anastomotic stoma (Fig. 6.17).

Postoperative DSA showed the patency of the reimplanted PICA (arrow) and obliteration of the aneurysm (Fig. 6.18).

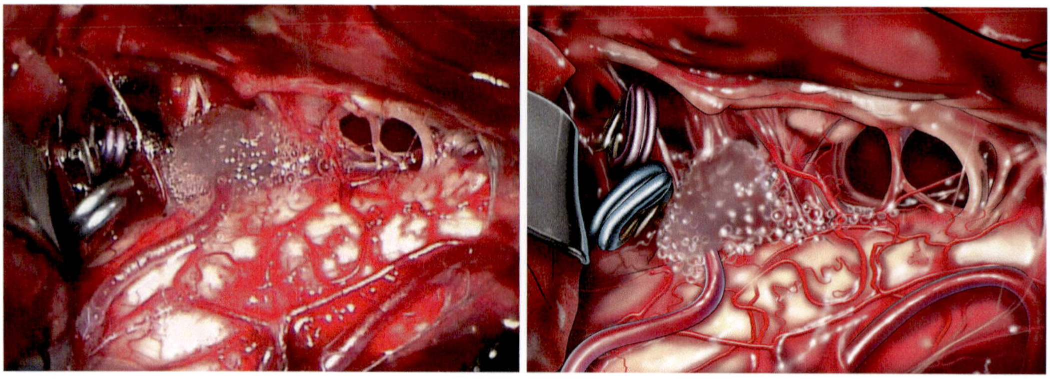

Fig. 6.17 The temporary clips were removed to check for oozing from the anastomotic stoma, and additional stitches were placed to stop the bleeding, if necessary. A Doppler probe was used to confirm the patency of the PICA. Surgicel and bioglue were applied to reinforce the anastomotic stoma

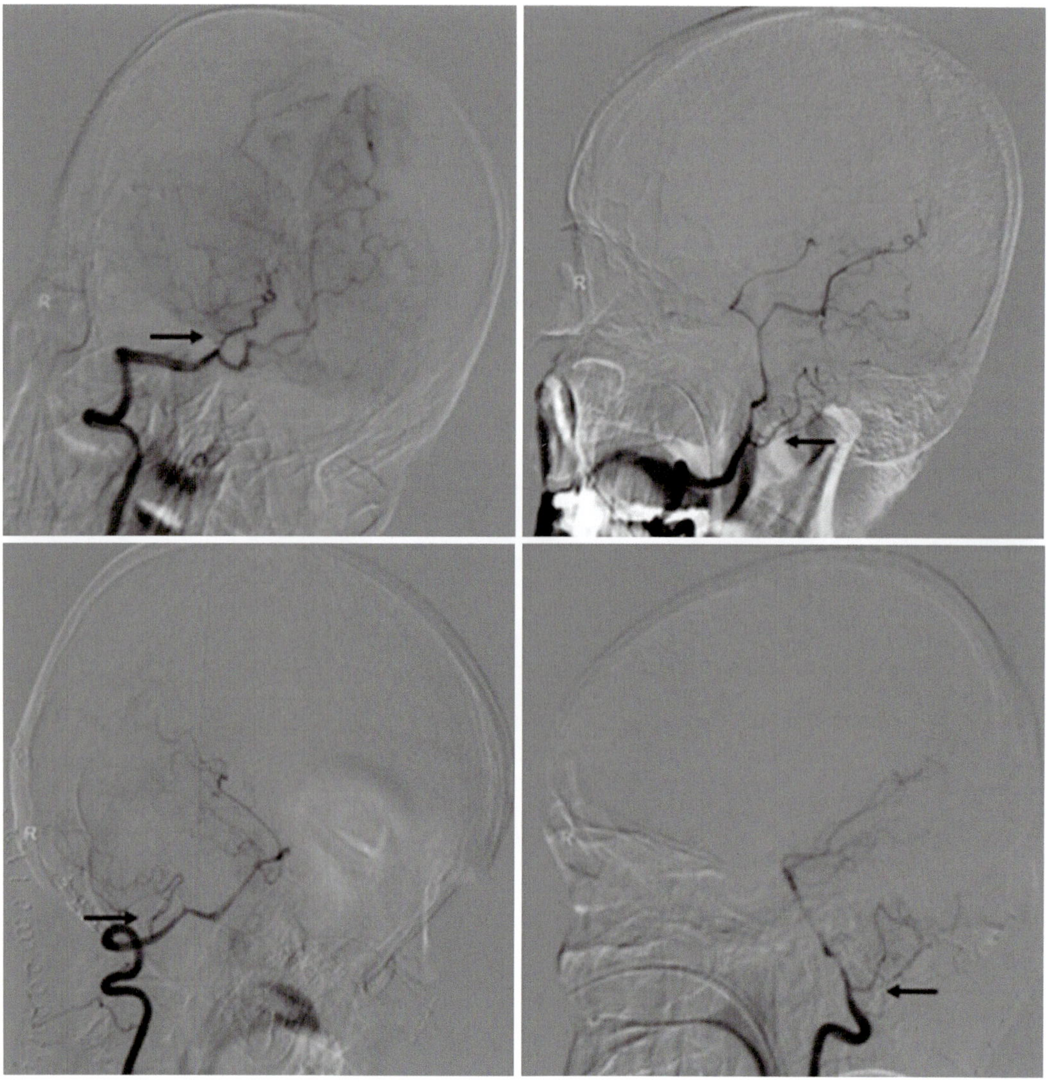

Fig. 6.18 Postoperative DSA showed the patency of the reimplanted PICA (arrow) and obliteration of the aneurysm

6.4 Comment

Because there is a collateral supply to the basilar circulation from the contralateral VA, this vessel may be more tolerant to prolonged temporary occlusion than the internal carotid artery. Therefore, a balloon test occlusion (BOT) is usually not needed before the bypass.

One of the challenges of PICA-VA bypass is that the V4 is usually trapped by the intertwined fragile cranial nerves. However, if the V4 is long enough, temporary clips could be placed between the nerves, leaving a 5–10 mm length of the V4 as the recipient artery. Atherosclerotic disease of the VA wall may raise the anastomotic stoma occlusion risk [2].

Another concern is that if the presence of direct medullary perforators from the proximal PICA are detected, PICA-VA reimplantation should be halted and replaced by other techniques, such as PICA-PICA bypass or OA-PICA bypass.

References

1. Sanai N, Zador Z, Lawton MT. Bypass surgery for complex brain aneurysms: an assessment of intracranial-intracranial bypass. Neurosurgery. 2009;65(4):670–83. 683
2. Abla AA, McDougall CM, Breshears JD, Lawton MT. Intracranial-to-intracranial bypass for posterior inferior cerebellar artery aneurysms: options, technical challenges, and results in 35 patients. J Neurosurg. 2016;124(5):1275–86.

Posterior Cerebral Artery-Posterior Cerebral Artery Bypass

7

Qi Yue, Xiaowen Wang, and Wei Zhu

Abstract

Reconstruction of posterior cerebral artery (PCA) could be performed with superficial temporal artery-PCA (STA-PCA) bypass, in situ PCA-superior cerebellar artery (PCA-SCA) bypass, or P2-P2 reanastomosis. The PCA and SCA are anatomically parallel; however, the PCA caliber is typically double that of the SCA, which limits the utility of PCA-SCA bypass. When treating some complex P2 aneurysms, end-to-end P2-P2 reanastomosis could be performed directly. However, due to the small redundancy and tortuosity of the PCA, it is difficult to perform end-to-end reanastomosis after resection of a giant aneurysm.

Here, we present a case of a previously coiled large PCA aneurysm that was treated by direct end-to-end bypass.

Keywords

Intracranial aneurysm · Intracranial-intracranial bypass · Posterior cerebral artery Reanastomosis · Revascularization bypass

Q. Yue · X. Wang · W. Zhu (✉)
Huashan Hospital, Shanghai Medical College, Fudan University, Shanghai, China
e-mail: drzhuwei@fudan.edu.cn

7.1 Introduction

Only 1% of intracranial aneurysms affect the posterior cerebral artery (PCA) [1, 2]. Cerebral revascularization of the PCA is effective in treating PCA lesions, especially some complex cerebral aneurysms.

There are several choices for PCA revascularization. When treating aneurysms in the P1 segment of the PCA, the posterior communicating artery (PcoA) reduces the need for bypass. The PcoA could be proximally occluded or trapped and provides the distal P2 blood supply. Evaluating the PcoA diameter and blood supply sufficiency is necessary for P1 aneurysms and decides whether bypass is needed. For P2 aneurysms, the abundant collateral blood supply provides a chance for direct PCA occlusion. A balloon occlusion test (BOT) is needed to assess the ischemia tolerance of the occipital lobe.

Reconstruction of PCA could be performed with superficial temporal artery-PCA (STA-PCA) bypass, in situ PCA-superior cerebellar artery (PCA-SCA) bypass, or P2-P2 reanastomosis. The PCA and SCA are anatomically parallel; however, the PCA caliber is typically double that of the SCA, which limits the utility of PCA-SCA bypass. When treating some complex P2 aneurysms, end-to-end P2-P2 reanastomosis could be performed directly. However, due to the small redundancy and tortuosity of the PCA, it is diffi-

Y. Mao et al. (eds.), *Surgical Atlas of Cerebral Revascularization*,
https://doi.org/10.1007/978-981-16-0374-7_7

cult to perform end-to-end reanastomosis after resection of a giant aneurysm.

The approaches to PCA varied from anterior to posterior, including pterional approach, transpetrosal approach, and occipital interhemispheric approach [3–5].

7.2 Case

A 55-year-old woman presented with blurry vision and ptosis in the right eye for 2 months. The preoperative physical examination showed that her vision field was normal, with VOD 0.4, VOS 0.8, and right oculomotor nerve palsy. She was diagnosed with a right PCA aneurysm and was treated by embolization 3 years ago. Preoperative head computed tomography (CT), high-resolution magnetic resonance imaging (MRI), and digital subtraction angiography (DSA) showed recurrence of the right PCA aneurysm (Fig. 7.1).

Retreatment by endovascular coiling was not applicable this time. Therefore, aneurysm resection with direct end-to-end PCA-PCA bypass was the first choice for this patient (Fig. 7.2). The STA was considered an alternative bypass donor.

7.3 Details of the Procedure

The operation was carried out in a hybrid operation suite. During the operation, the patient was placed in the supine position with a headholder, and a right orbitozygomatic craniotomy was performed. After opening the dura, a small piece of the temporal pole was resected to expose the recurrent PCA aneurysm. The coils could be seen inside the aneurysm, and the aneurysm had tight adhesions to nearby structures (Fig. 7.3).

Because of the high tension of the aneurysm body, gaining proximal control was difficult. Therefore, after catheterization of the femoral artery, a 5F guiding catheter was placed into the right vertebral artery, and the P1 segment of the right PCA was blocked by a Gateway balloon. The right P2 segment was temporarily blocked with a clip. With the assistance of interrupted

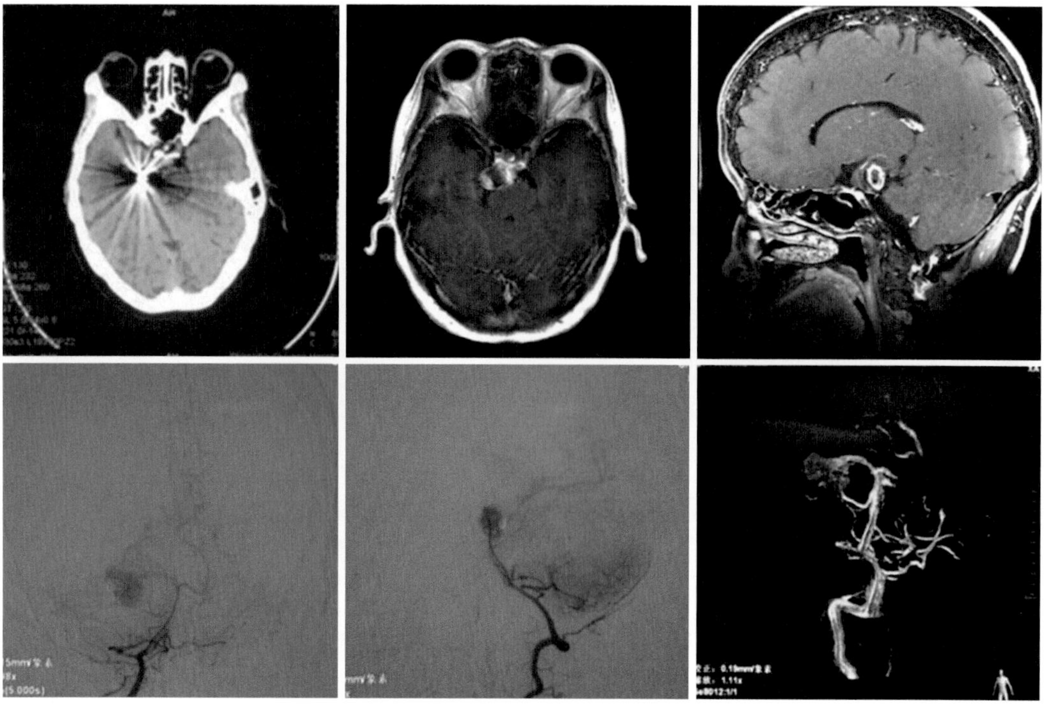

Fig. 7.1 Preoperative head CT, high-resolution MRI, and DSA showed recurrence of the right PCA aneurysm

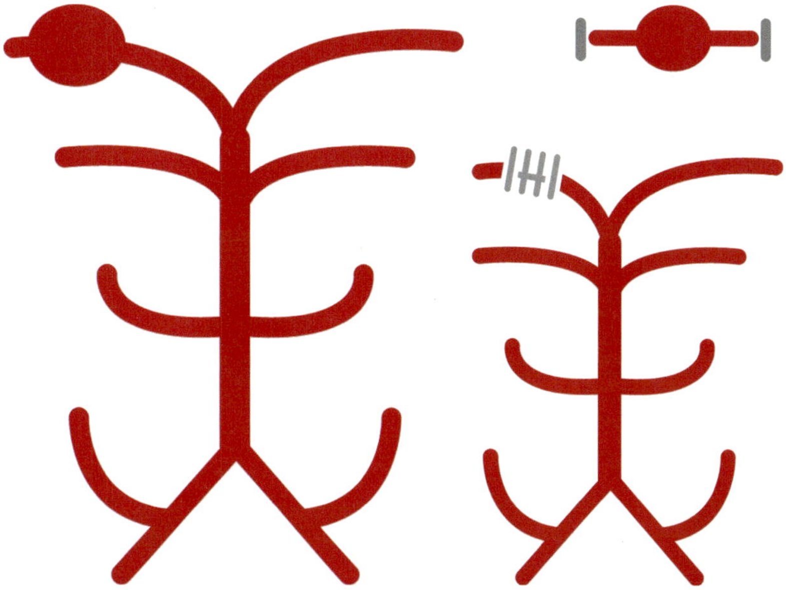

Fig. 7.2 Surgical plan: PCA aneurysm resection with direct end-to-end PCA-PCA bypass

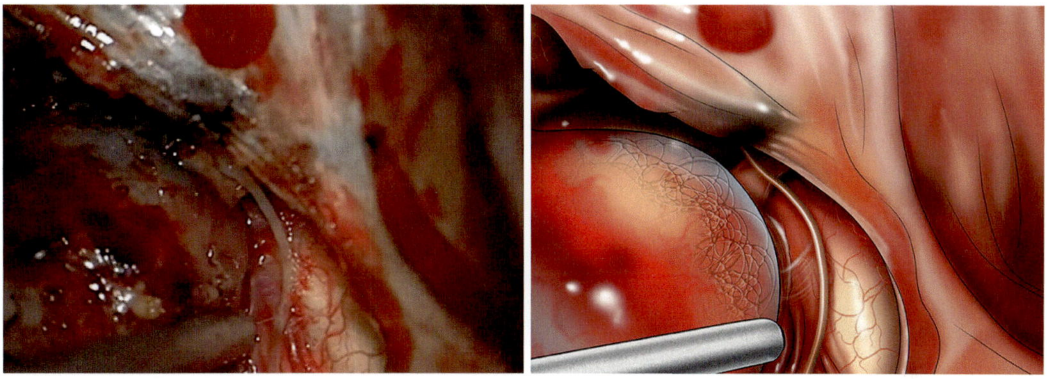

Fig. 7.3 After performing orbitozygomatic craniotomy and opening the dura, a small piece of the temporal pole was resected to expose the recurrent PCA aneurysm

releases and inflations of the Gateway balloon, the tension of the aneurysm decreased, and the adhesions around the aneurysm were separated. When the P2 segment proximal to the aneurysm could be exposed, a temporary clip was placed, and the balloon was withdrawn (Fig. 7.4).

The aneurysm was resected piece by piece, and the inflow tract (proximal P2) and outflow tract (distal P2) were released from the adhesions and trimmed (Fig. 7.5). The lumina was flushed with heparinized saline, and the intima edges were marked by methylene blue. An end-to-end anastomosis strategy was applied for the proximal P2 and distal P2 (Fig. 7.6). The first suture was placed at the bottom of the anastomotic stoma (Fig. 7.7), and the second suture was placed at the top of the anastomotic stoma (Fig. 7.8). A total of 3–5 interrupted sutures were placed at each edge of the anastomotic stoma (Figs. 7.9 and 7.10). After the anastomosis was complete, the temporary clips were removed in a distal to proximal direction (Fig. 7.11).

Intraoperative indocyanine green angiography confirmed patency of the anastomosis (Fig. 7.12).

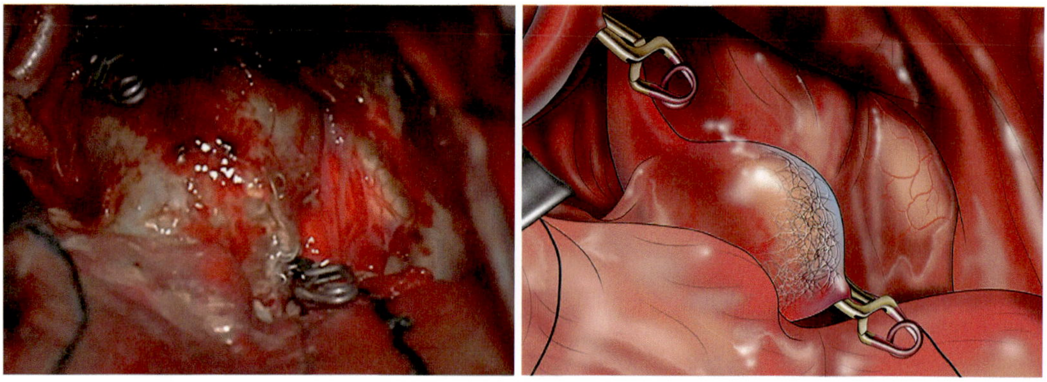

Fig. 7.4 The P1 segment of the right PCA was blocked by a Gateway balloon. The right P2 segment was temporarily blocked with a clip. With the assistance of interrupted releases and inflations of the Gateway balloon, the tension of the aneurysm decreased, and the adhesions around the aneurysm were separated. When the P2 segment proximal to the aneurysm could be exposed, a temporary clip was placed, and the balloon was withdrawn

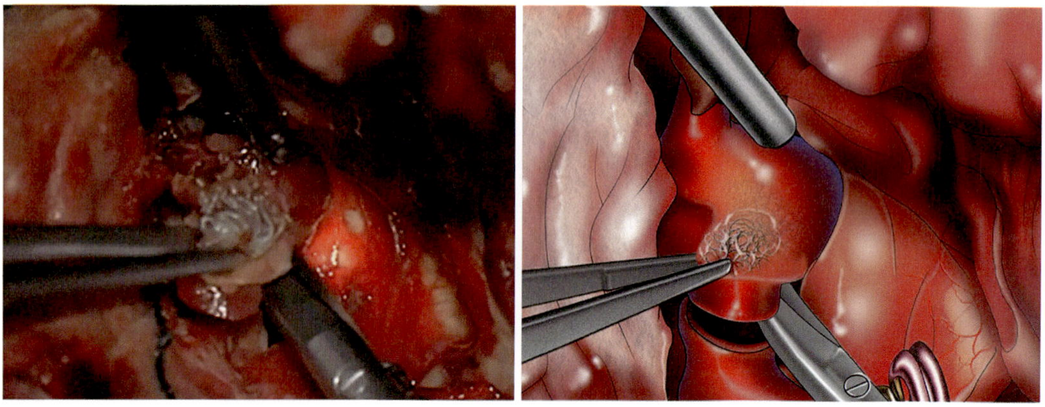

Fig. 7.5 The aneurysm was resected piece by piece, and the inflow and outflow tracts of the aneurysm were carefully trimmed

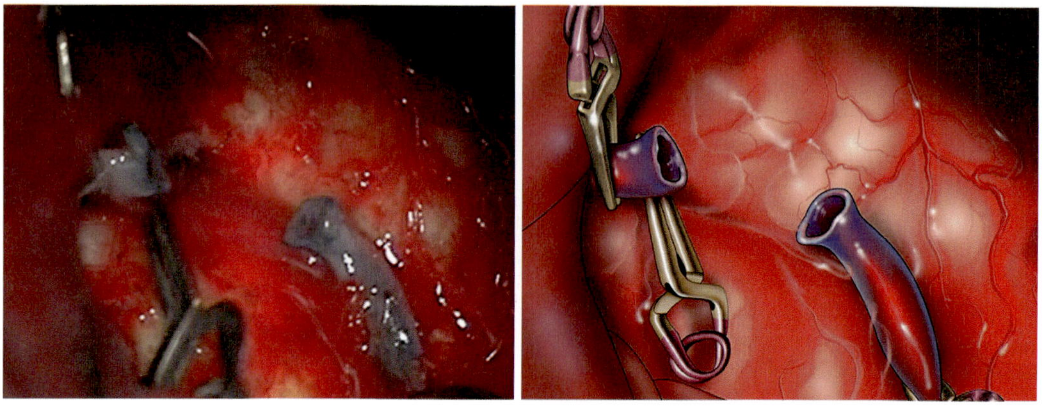

Fig. 7.6 An end-to-end anastomosis strategy was applied for the inflow tract (proximal P2) and outflow tract (distal P2) of the aneurysm. The proximal P2 and distal P2 were released from the adhesions and trimmed. Then, the lumina was flushed with heparinized saline, and the intima edges were marked by methylene blue

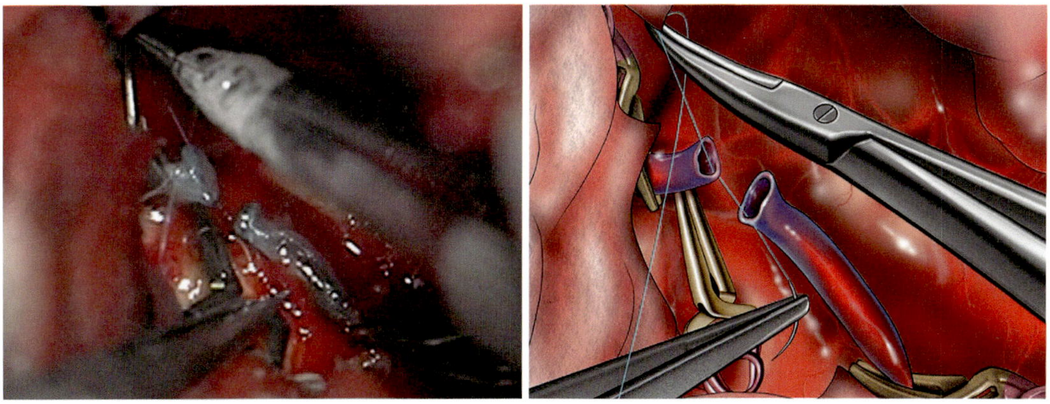

Fig. 7.7 The first suture was placed at the bottom of the anastomotic stoma

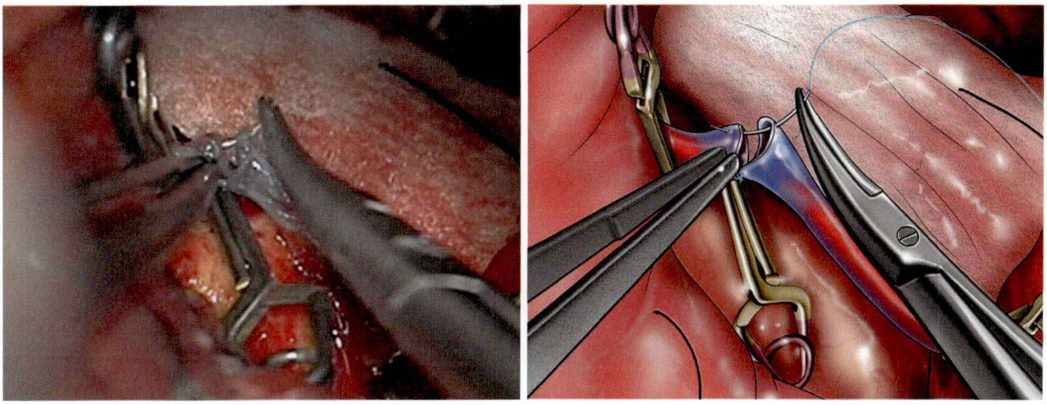

Fig. 7.8 The second suture was placed at the top of the anastomotic stoma

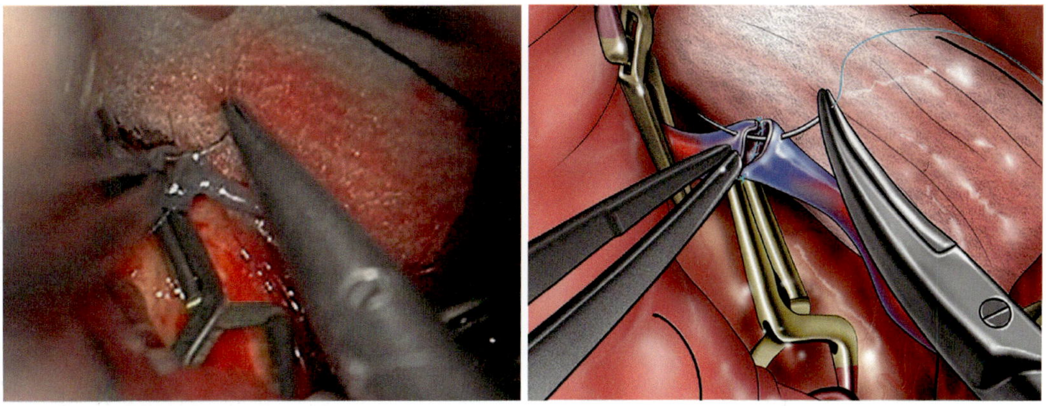

Fig. 7.9 One edge of the anastomotic stoma was sutured with 3–5 interrupted stitches

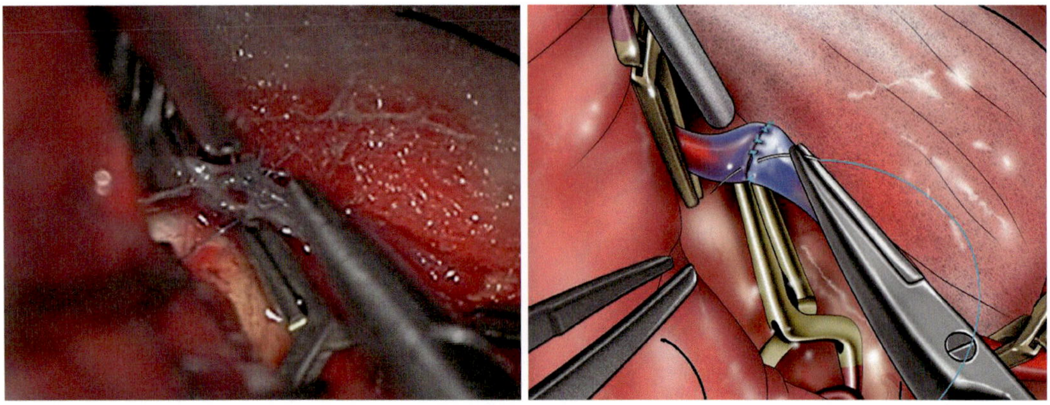

Fig. 7.10 The other edge of the anastomotic stoma was also sutured with 3–5 interrupted stitches

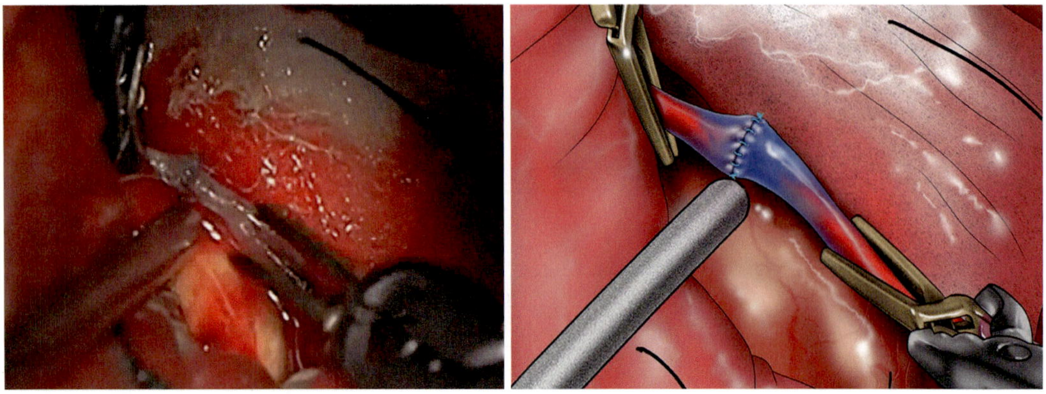

Fig. 7.11 After the anastomosis was complete, the temporary clips were removed in a distal to proximal direction

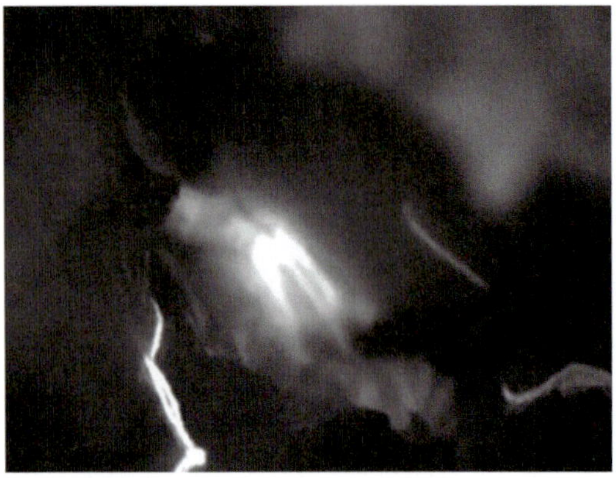

Fig. 7.12 Intraoperative indocyanine green angiography confirmed patency of the anastomosis

7.4 Comment

This case showed the surgical treatment of a complex recurrent aneurysm that was coiled 3 years ago. Interventional therapy was not applicable for retreatment. Although direct PCA occlusion with coils was reported to be relatively safe, the elevated risk of distal PCA region infarction could not be ignored [6–9]. Because there is sufficient collateral flow from the leptomeningeal region, BOT is sometimes unreliable. Cerebral revascularization was a better choice for this PCA aneurysm.

Sundt showed the first PCA bypass case in 1982 [10]. Lawton showed that different bypass strategies for PCA lesions can be used in different situations according to PcoA diameter and BOT with hypotensive challenge [11]. In situ PCA bypasses are feasible when clipping cannot preserve flow in the P1 segment of the PCA, the PcoA is diminutive or occluded, or the STA is also diminutive or unavailable [12]. PCA-occipital artery (OA) bypass is also used in some cases. However, the OA tapers above the superior nuchal line and may have an insufficient diameter and length [13].

When choosing an approach to the PCA, both the anastomosed portion of the PCA and the bypass strategy should be taken into consideration. Anterior approaches, including the pterional approach without opening the sylvian fissure and the anterior temporal approach (ATA), expose the P1, PcoA, and anterior portion of P2. The lateral approaches include the subtemporal approach, lateral ATA, extradural subtemporal approach, subtemporal approach combined with an anterior transpetrosal approach, combined transpetrosal approach, and partial mastoidectomy. These approaches aim to expose the P2 and posterior P2 segments. The reported posterior approaches include the infraoccipital supratentorial approach, supracerebellar infratentorial approach, and posterior interhemispheric approach, aiming to expose the posterior P2, P3, and far distal P4 segments [14, 15].

This surgery was performed in a hybrid operating room. Performing craniotomy in combination with intervention provided a safer way to gain proximal control of the aneurysm, perform resection and confirm patency of the bypass.

References

1. Honda M, Tsutsumi K, Yokoyama H, Yonekura M, Nagata I. Aneurysms of the posterior cerebral artery: retrospective review of surgical treatment. Neurol Med Chir (Tokyo). 2004;44(4):164–8. 169
2. Locksley HB. Natural history of subarachnoid hemorrhage, intracranial aneurysms and arteriovenous malformations. Based on 6368 cases in the cooperative study. J Neurosurg. 1966;25(2):219–39.
3. Goehre F, Kamiyama H, Noda K, Ota N, Tsuboi T, Miyata S, Matsumoto T, Yanagisawa T, Tokuda S, Tanikawa R. Technical Description of the Medial and Lateral Anterior Temporal Approach for the Treatment of Complex Proximal Posterior Cerebral Artery Aneurysms. World Neurosurg. 2016;86:490–6.
4. Ota N, Tanikawa R, Eda H, Matsumoto T, Miyazaki T, Matsukawa H, Yanagisawa T, Suzuki G, Miyata S, Oda J, Noda K, Tsuboi T, Takeda R, Kamiyama H, Tokuda S. Radical treatment for bilateral vertebral artery dissecting aneurysms by reconstruction of the vertebral artery. J Neurosurg. 2016;125(4):953–63.
5. Tayebi MA, Lawton MT, Griswold D, Mokhtari P, Payman A, Tabani H, Yousef S, Benet A. Revascularization of the upper posterior circulation with the anterior temporal artery: an anatomical feasibility study. J Neurosurg. 2018;129(1):121–7.
6. Jayakumar PN, Desai S, Srikanth SG, Ravishankar S, Kovoor JM. Relevance of occlusion test in endovascular coiling of posterior cerebral artery (p2 segment) aneurysms. Interv Neuroradiol. 2004;10(3):235–48.
7. Arat A, Islak C, Saatci I, Kocer N, Cekirge S. Endovascular parent artery occlusion in large-giant or fusiform distal posterior cerebral artery aneurysms. Neuroradiology. 2002;44(8):700–5.
8. Ciceri EF, Klucznik RP, Grossman RG, Rose JE, Mawad ME. Aneurysms of the posterior cerebral artery: classification and endovascular treatment. AJNR Am J Neuroradiol. 2001;22(1):27–34.
9. Cotroneo E, Gigli R, Guglielmi G. Endovascular occlusion of the posterior cerebral artery in the treatment of p2 ruptured aneurysms. Interv Neuroradiol. 2007;13(2):127–32.
10. Sundt TJ, Piepgras DG, Houser OW, Campbell JK. Interposition saphenous vein grafts for advanced occlusive disease and large aneurysms in the posterior circulation. J Neurosurg. 1982;56(2):205–15.
11. Lawton M. Seven Bypasses. Thieme: Tenets and Techniques for Revascularization; 2018.
12. Quinones-Hinojosa A, Lawton MT. In situ bypass in the management of complex intracranial aneurysms: technique application in 13 patients. Neurosurgery. 2005;57(1 Suppl):140–5. 140-45
13. Keser N, Avci E, Soylemez B, Karatas D, Baskaya MK. Occipital Artery and Its Segments in Vertebral Artery Revascularization Surgery: A Microsurgical Anatomic Study. World Neurosurg. 2018;112:e534–9.
14. Ota N, Goehre F, Miyazaki T, Kinoshita Y, Matsukawa H, Yanagisawa T, Sakakibara F, Saito N, Miyata S, Noda K, Tsuboi T, Kamiyama H, Tokuda S, Kamada K, Tanikawa R. Bypass Revascularization Applied to the Posterior Cerebral Artery. World Neurosurg. 2016;96:460–72.
15. Tanahashi K, Araki Y, Uda K, Muraoka S, Motomura K, Lushun C, Wakabayashi T, Natsume A. Posterior Cerebral Artery Reconstruction by In-Situ Bypass with Superior Cerebellar Artery via Occipital Transtentorial Approach. World Neurosurg. 2019;126:24–9.

8 Anterior Cerebral Artery-Anterior Cerebral Artery Bypass

Peiliang Li, Qingzhu An, and Wei Zhu

Abstract

The anterior cerebral artery (ACA) can be defined as two main parts by the anterior communicating artery (ACoA): the horizontal part/the precommunicating segment and the vertical part/the postcommunicating segment. The bilateral ACAs run in parallel in the interhemispheric fissure beyond the ACoA, providing the advantage of an intracranial (IC)-IC bypass pattern to aid the other if one is occluded or has to be sacrificed. There are various technical options for ACA revascularization, including reanastomosis, in situ bypass, reimplantation, and bypass with short interposition grafts.

Here, we present a case of a large recurrent ACA A1 segment aneurysm with poor compensating ACoA blood flow that was treated by an ACA A3-A3 in situ bypass combined with A1 parent artery coiling.

Keywords

Anterior cerebral artery · Anterior communicating artery · In situ bypass · Intracranial aneurysm · Intracranial-intracranial bypass Revascularization

P. Li · Q. An · W. Zhu (✉)
Huashan Hospital, Shanghai Medical College, Fudan University, Shanghai, China
e-mail: drzhuwei@fudan.edu.cn

8.1 Introduction

The anterior cerebral artery (ACA) can be defined as two main parts by the anterior communicating artery (ACoA): the horizontal part/the precommunicating segment and the vertical part/the postcommunicating segment. The bilateral ACAs run in parallel in the interhemisphere fissure beyond the ACoA, providing the advantage of an intracranial (IC)-IC bypass pattern to aid the other if one is occluded or has to be sacrificed. There are various technical options for ACA revascularization, including reanastomosis, in situ bypass, reimplantation, and bypass with short interposition grafts.

Here, we present a case of a large recurrent ACA A1 segment aneurysm with poor compensating ACoA blood flow that was treated by an ACA A3-A3 in situ bypass combined with A1 parent artery coiling.

8.2 Case

A 28-year-old woman suffered from sudden headache and vomiting one day prior. Physical examination before the operation showed that her Glasgow coma score was 15, with neck stiffness and a positive Kernig sign. No neurological deficit was present, so the Hunt-Hess score was grade 2. Preoperative head computed tomography (CT) showed subarachnoid ventricular hemorrhage.

Y. Mao et al. (eds.), *Surgical Atlas of Cerebral Revascularization*,
https://doi.org/10.1007/978-981-16-0374-7_8

Digital subtraction angiography (DSA) showed a left ACA A1 segment aneurysm, and then the aneurysm was cured by stent-assisted coil embolization. Postoperative DSA showed that the aneurysm was embolized satisfactorily without obvious residue, and the parent artery was unobstructed. DSA reexamination was performed 3 months later and showed recurrence of the A1 segment aneurysm. Retreatment, such as stent-assisted aneurysm embolization or surgical clipping, could not be applied in this case. A balloon occlusion test of the ipsilateral internal carotid artery (ICA) was undertaken, and the results showed that the ACoA had poor compensation (Fig. 8.1). Therefore, we planned to perform A3-A3 bypass and then occlude the left A1 by coiling (Fig. 8.2).

8.3 Details of the Procedure

During the operation, the patient was placed supine in a head holder, and a right frontal curved incision crossing the midline was made. After craniotomy with a 6 cm × 6 cm bone window, the superior sagittal sinus was exposed. The dura was opened, and the anterior interhemispheric fissure was carefully dissected under a microscope. The bilateral A3 segments of the ACA were exposed (Fig. 8.3).

A side-to-side anastomosis was applied to the bilateral A3 segment bypass. At first, both arteries were occluded temporarily; then, the anastomotic sites on the bilateral A3 segments were cut open in a linear fashion, and the length of the incision was approximately 2 times the diameter

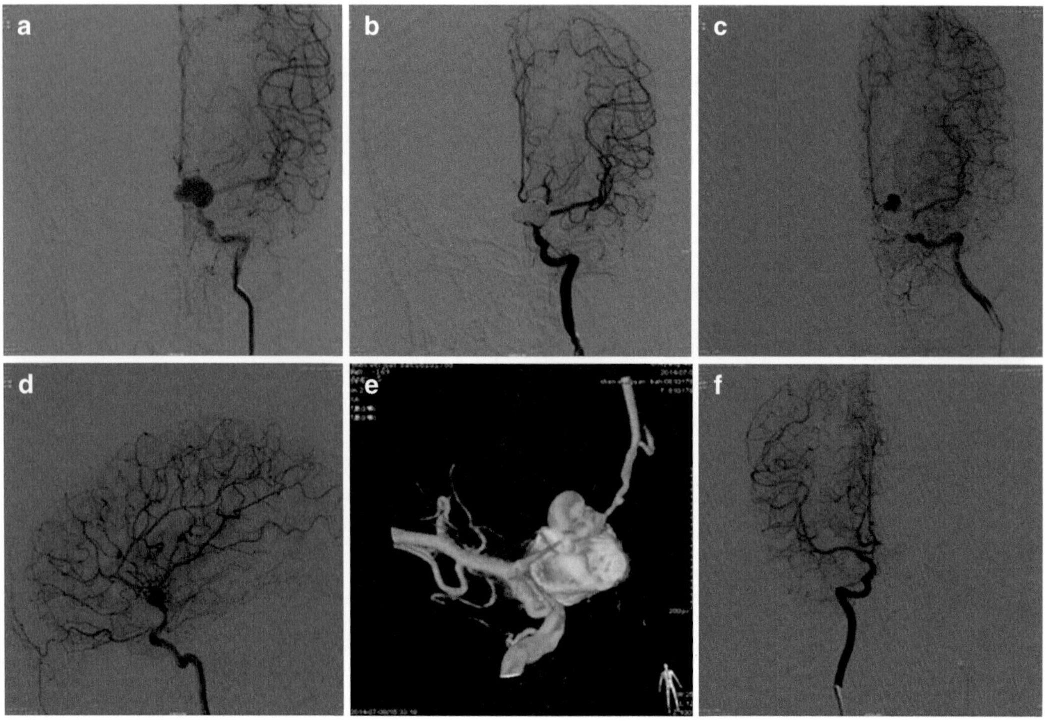

Fig. 8.1 (**a**) Preoperative DSA showed a large aneurysm of the left A1 segment; (**b**) After endovascular therapy, DSA showed that the aneurysm was embolized satisfactorily without obvious residue, and the parent artery was unobstructed; (**c**, **d**, **e**) DSA reexamination was performed 3 months later, and the results showed recurrence of the A1 segment aneurysm; (**f**) A balloon occlusion test of the ipsilateral ICA was undertaken, and the results showed that the ACoA had poor compensation

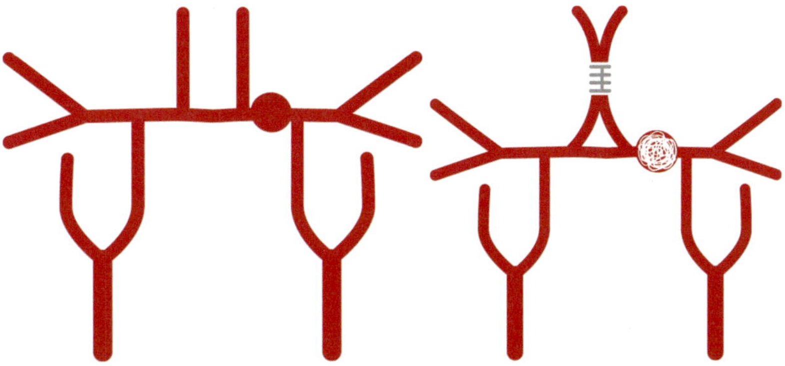

Fig. 8.2 Surgical plan: A3-A3 bypass and left A1 occlusion by coiling

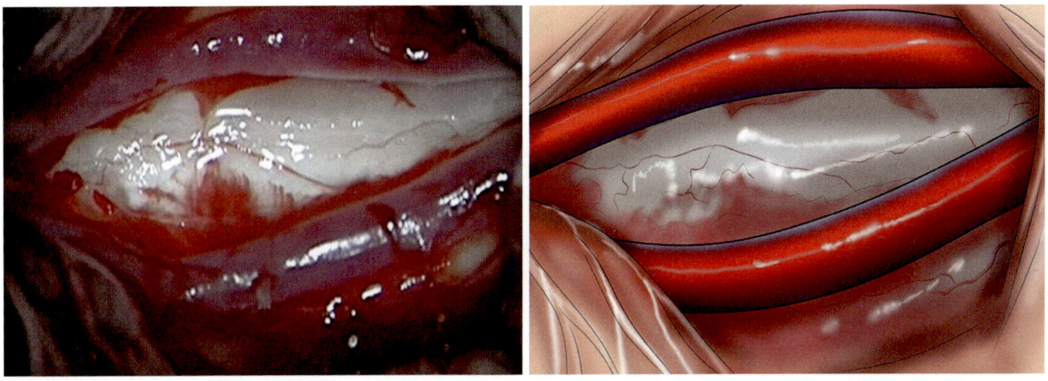

Fig. 8.3 The anterior interhemispheric fissure was carefully dissected under a microscope. The bilateral A3 segments of the ACA were exposed

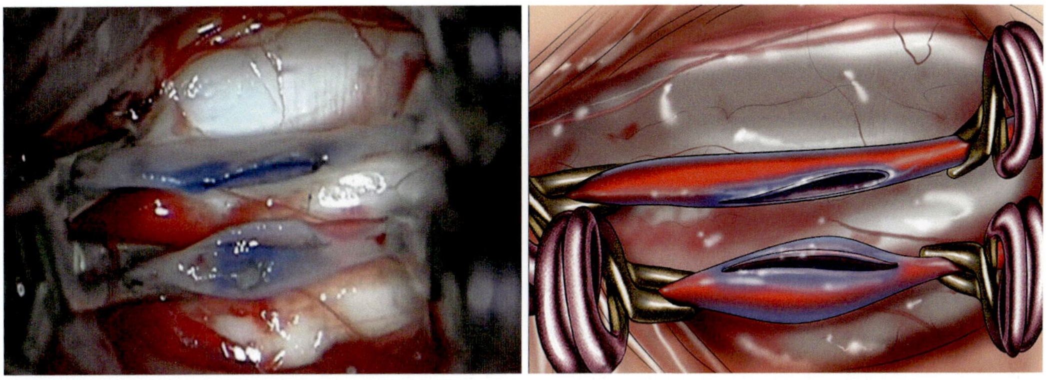

Fig. 8.4 A side-to-side anastomosis was applied to the bilateral A3 segment bypass. At first, both arteries were occluded temporarily; then, the anastomotic sites on the bilateral A3 segments were cut open in a linear fashion, and the length of the incision was approximately 2 times the diameter of the vessel

of the vessel (Fig. 8.4). The artery lumina were flushed with heparinized saline, and the edges of the anastomotic sites were marked with methylene blue. The anastomosis started at the posterior wall of the anastomotic stoma. The knot of the first stitch was placed outside the artery, and the second stitch was placed from the outside to the inside of the artery wall. Then, suturing was carried out continuously (Fig. 8.5). When the continuous suturing of the posterior wall was

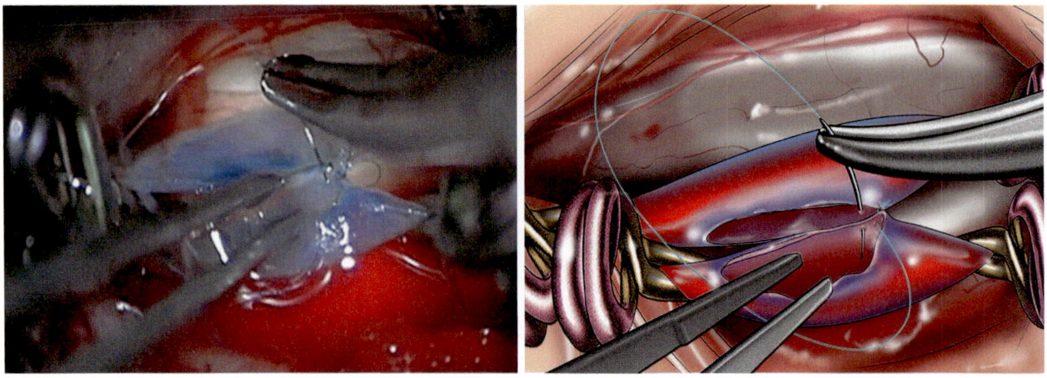

Fig. 8.5 The anastomosis started at the posterior wall of the anastomotic stoma. The knot of the first stitch was placed outside the artery, and the second stitch was placed from the outside to the inside of the artery wall. Then, suturing was carried out continuously

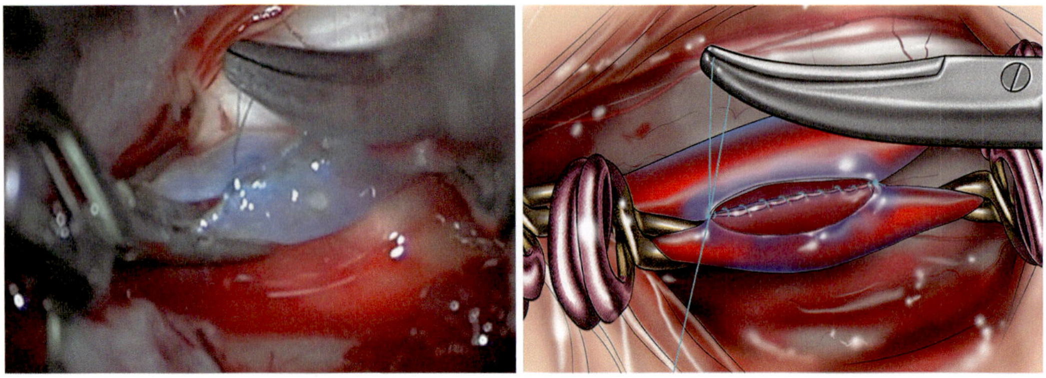

Fig. 8.6 When the continuous suturing of the posterior wall was completed at the other end of the stoma, the knot of the final stitch was tied outside the artery

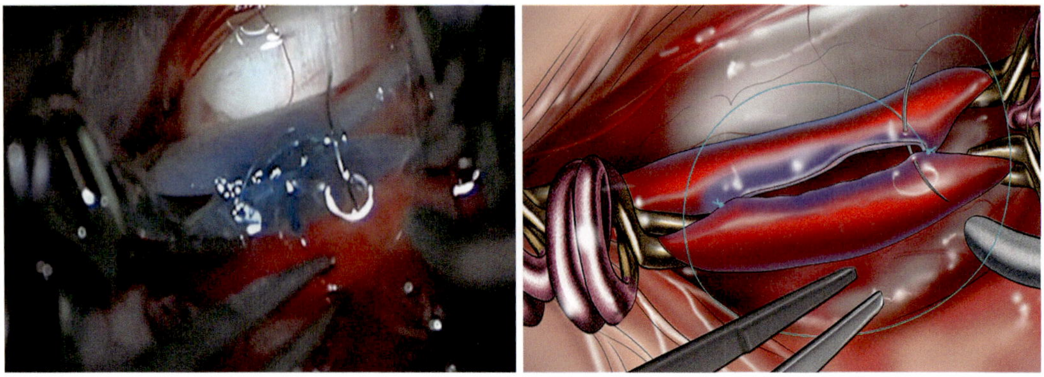

Fig. 8.7 Similarly, the anterior wall of the anastomotic stoma was also continuously sutured

completed at the other end of the stoma, the knot of the final stitch was tied outside the artery (Fig. 8.6). Similarly, the anterior wall of the anastomotic stoma was also continuously sutured (Fig. 8.7). After the anastomosis was completed, all temporary clips were removed. The stoma was

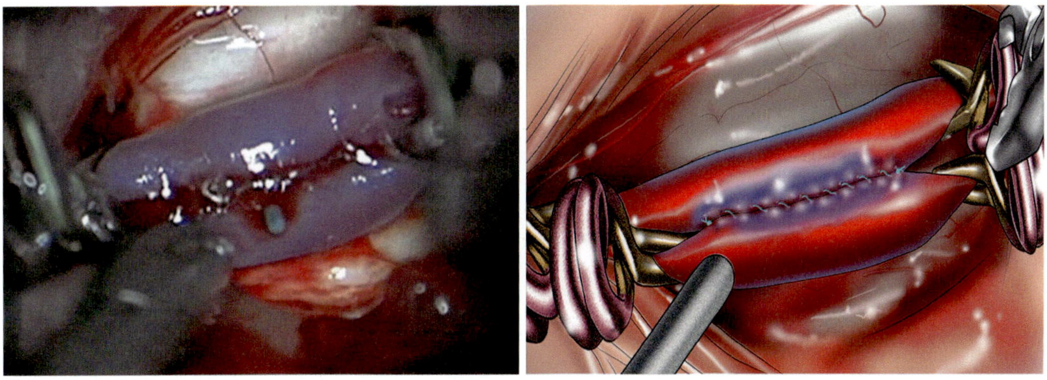

Fig. 8.8 After the anastomosis was completed, all temporary clips were removed. The stoma was inspected carefully to ensure that there was no oozing or stenosis

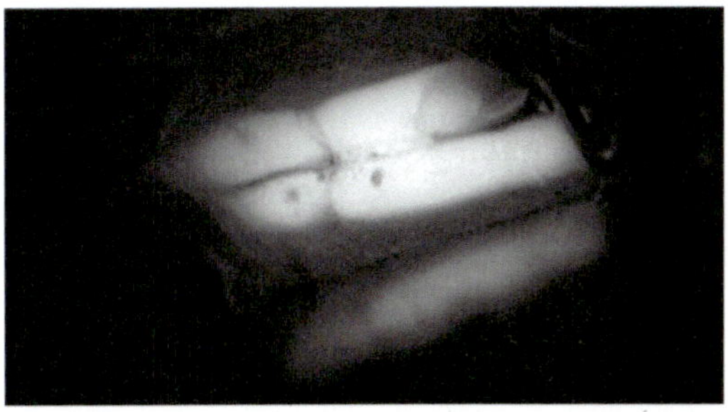

Fig. 8.9 Intraoperative indocyanine green angiography showed patency of the A3-A3 side-to-side bypass

inspected carefully to ensure that there was no oozing or stenosis (Fig. 8.8).

Intraoperative indocyanine green angiography showed patency of the A3-A3 side-to-side bypass (Fig. 8.9). Postoperative DSA performed the next day showed patency of the anastomosis, and the volume of the aneurysm had significantly decreased. Therefore, we did not occlude the parent A1 artery immediately due to the possibility of aneurysm self-healing. However, follow-up DSA performed 10 days later showed enlargement of the aneurysm, so we performed parent A1 artery occlusion. After endovascular embolization of the parent artery and aneurysm, ipsilateral ICA angiography showed that the left A1 segment was occluded and the aneurysm had disappeared. Contralateral ICA angiography showed patency of the anastomosis, that the blood flow of the ipsilateral A2 segment was reversed, and the aneurysm was not displayed (Fig. 8.10).

8.4 Comment

ACA-ACA side-to-side in situ anastomosis is the most reasonable and most straightforward option for reconstructing the blood flow of the ACA, especially in the case of complex aneurysms involving the ACoA complex or its branches, although these aneurysms are relatively rare in the clinic. This type of anastomosis was first described and published in 1980 by Ito [1]. In situ bypass may be performed anywhere along with the distal ACA. However, the sizeable arterial caliber and accessibility of the distal A2 segments at the top of the rostrum and A3 at the genu make them favorable sites for side-to-side bypass [2]. However, this operation is one of the most technically difficult bypasses because it has to be performed in a very narrow corridor at a depth of 6–8 cm [3], and sutures of the deep edge of the anastomosis need to be performed in an irregular side-to-outside pattern, which demands an experienced neurosurgeon [4]. Several techniques can facilitate the procedure of this bypass [2, 5]. The supine position is usually utilized for in situ A3-A3 side-by-side bypass. The anterior frontal lobe tends to fall laterally and inferiorly due to gravity retraction. The lumbar drainage, anesthetic, and osmotic brain relaxation maneuvers are helpful to increase the vessel exposure and avoid long-time fixed retraction. The sizeable superficial bridging veins encountered in the interhemispheric access to the A3 ACA should be

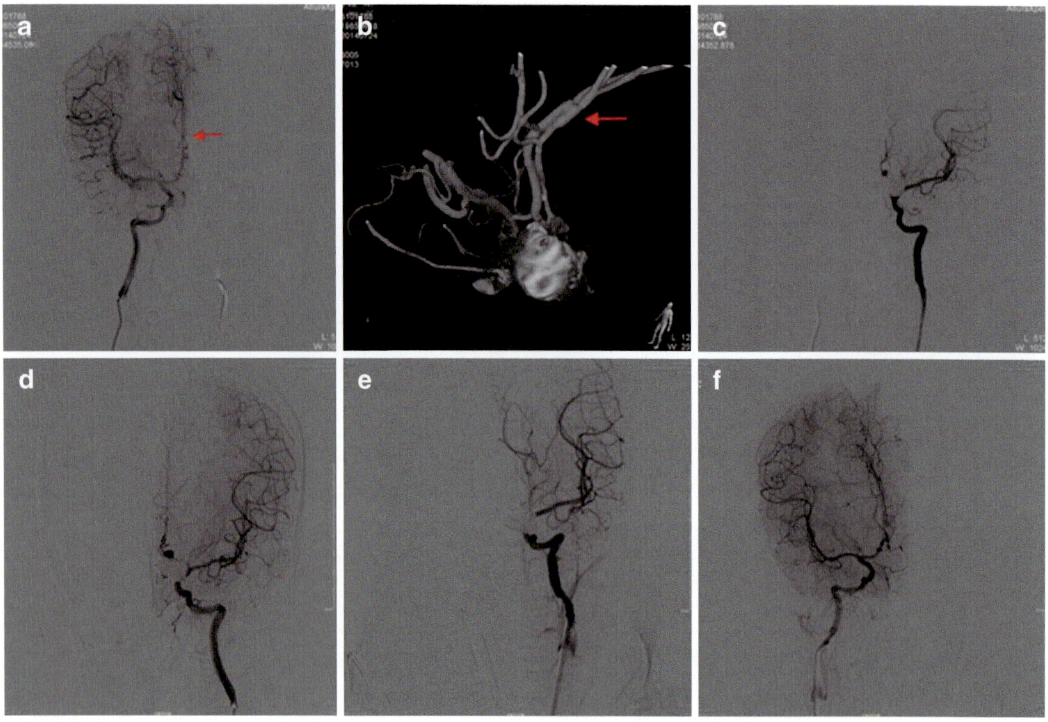

Fig. 8.10 (**a**, **b**) Postoperative DSA showed patency of the anastomosis (red arrow); (**c**) The volume of the aneurysm significantly decreased; (**d**) Follow-up DSA 10 days later showed enlargement of the aneurysm; (**e**, **f**) After endovascular embolization of the parent artery and aneurysm, ipsilateral ICA angiography showed that the left A1 segment was occluded and the aneurysm had disappeared. Contralateral ICA angiography showed patency of the anastomosis, that the blood flow of the ipsilateral A2 segment was reversed, and the aneurysm was not displayed

sharply dissected and protected by wrapping in Surgicel and fibrin glue. The ribbon retractors against the falx can be used. However, if the A3 exposure is still limited, the ipsilateral hemisphere's retraction may be applied with caution. The vessels for bypass must be fully released and mobilized from the arachnoid membrane. A rubber dam, along with a small piece of gelfoam downside, is placed beneath both vessels. This maneuver can isolate and elevate the vessels for better manipulation. We suggest arteriotomies better be placed at roughly the 2 o'clock and 10 o'clock positions on both vessels' medial aspects for best visibility inside the lumen. Therefore, the arteriotomies margins are optimally apposed for both front- and back-wall sutures.

There are three other different IC-IC bypass patterns for ACA blood flow reconstruction: reanastomosis, reimplantation, and interposition graft bypass [6–8]. If a hypoplastic or aplastic contralateral A1 is identified, the ipsilateral A1 can be reconstructed using reanastomosis in an end-to-end fashion, or end-to-end/end-to-side bypass with a short interposition graft [9]. However, reanastomosis is the least common IC-IC reconstructive technique. The little redundancy after aneurysm excision brings difficulty in reapproximating the arterial stump [10].

ACA reimplantation can be performed with both ipsilateral and contralateral variations [11]. Ipsilateral reimplantation is a vertical bypass, with the ipsilateral callosal marginal artery (CmaA) or pericallosal artery (PcaA) mobilized across the cingulate gyrus aggressively to get connected superoinferiorly. Contralateral reimplantation is a horizontal bypass, with the ACA, CmaA, or PcaA freed to get left-right connected. Reimplantation is a versatile technique. The ipsilateral efferent arteries that run parallel to uninvolved contralateral arteries might serve as donors (end-to-side left-right bypass) [12]. Besides, a left frontopolar artery-right A2 ACA bypass was reported by Spetzler et al. [13] for the treatment of a complex ACA pseudoaneurysm.

Lawton et al. [14] reported the "azygos bypass" technique. A RAG was used to build an azygos circulation from one A2 segment to the PcaA and CmaA on the other side in the interhemispheric fissure (left-right bypass). The STA is not applicable for the direct bypass to ACA because this lateral scalp artery may not reach efferent arteries deeply seated in the interhemispheric fissure. However, by using the contralateral STA as an interposition graft, STA-ACA bypass had been reported to treat complex ACA aneurysms successfully by Park et al. [4].

While IC-IC bypass has several advantages, such as the lack of need for additional flow, the lack of requirement for graft harvest and neck incision, and the use of only one anastomosis, IC-IC still has some limitations. In addition to the technical difficulties, there are two main limitations: (1) if bypass fails, the procedure can injure the two cerebral arteries; and (2) in the case of a more proximal vascular lesion, such as a precommunicating or communicating aneurysm, the procedure requires a combined craniotomy utilizing both interhemispheric and subfrontal corridors [15]. However, using a staged or hybrid endovascular aneurysm occlusion strategy, only a bifrontal-interhemispheric approach is sufficient, eliminating the need for combined craniotomy [16]. The anterior temporal artery (ATA) may be another choice for avoiding extended exposure. When ATA-ACA bypass is available, the aneurysm can be occluded after bypass in a single pterional craniotomy, obviating the interhemispheric exposure [17].

References

1. Ito Z. A new technique of intracranial interarterial anastomosis between distal anterior cerebral arteries (ACA) for ACA occlusion and its indication (author's transl). Neurol Med Chir (Tokyo). 1981;21(9):931–9.
2. Grigore FN, Amin-Hanjani S. A3-A3 bypass surgery for aneurysm: technical nuances. Oper Neurosurg (Hagerstown). 2019;17(3):277–85.
3. Hauck EF, Samson D. A1-A2 interposition grafting for surgical treatment of a giant "unclippable" A1 segment aneurysm. Surg Neurol. 2009;71(5):600–3.
4. Park ES, Ahn JS, Park JC, Kwon DH, Kwun BD, Kim CJ. STA-ACA bypass using the contralateral STA as an interposition graft for the treatment of complex ACA aneurysms: report of two cases and a review of the literature. Acta Neurochir. 2012;154(8):1447–53.
5. Abla AA, Lawton MT. Anterior cerebral artery bypass for complex aneurysms: an experience with intracranial-intracranial reconstruction and review of bypass options. J Neurosurg. 2014;120(6):1364–77.
6. Ewald CH, Kuhne D, Hassler WE. Bypass-surgery and coil-embolisation in the treatment of cerebral giant aneurysms. Acta Neurochir. 2000;142(7):731–7. 737-38
7. Gelfenbeyn M, Natarajan SK, Sekhar LN. Large distal anterior cerebral artery aneurysm treated with resection and interposition graft: case report. Neurosurgery. 2009;64(5):E1008–9. E1009
8. Sanai N, Zador Z, Lawton MT. Bypass surgery for complex brain aneurysms: an assessment of intracranial-intracranial bypass. Neurosurgery. 2009;65(4):670–83. 683
9. Endo H, Sugiyama SI, Endo T, Fujimura M, Shimizu H, Tominaga T. Revascularization of the anterior cerebral artery by Y-shaped superficial temporal artery interposition graft for the treatment of a de novo aneurysm arising at the site of A3-A3 bypass: technical case report. J Neurosurg. 2018;129(5):1120–4.
10. Matsushima K, Kawashima M, Suzuyama K, Takase Y, Takao T, Matsushima T. Thrombosed giant aneurysm of the distal anterior cerebral artery treated with aneurysm resection and proximal pericallosal artery-callosomarginal artery end-to-end anastomosis: case report and review of the literature. Surg Neurol Int. 2011;2:135.
11. Labib MA, Gandhi S, Cavallo C, Nisson PL, Mooney MA, Catapano JS, Lang MJ, Chen T, Lawton MT. Anterior cerebral artery bypass for complex aneurysms: advances in intracranial-intracranial bypass techniques. In: World Neurosurg, vol. 141; 2020. p. e42–54.
12. Yokoh A, Ausman JI, Dujovny M, Diaz FG, Berman SK, Sanders J, Mirchandani HG. Anterior cerebral artery reconstruction. Neurosurgery. 1986;19(1):26–35.
13. Chen PR, Abla AA, McDougall CG, Spetzler RF, Albuquerque FC. Surgical techniques for unclippable fusiform A2-anterior cerebral artery aneurysms and description of a frontopolar-to-A2 bypass. World Neurosurg. 2014;81(2):441–9.
14. Mirzadeh Z, Sanai N, Lawton MT. The azygos anterior cerebral artery bypass: double reimplantation technique for giant anterior communicating artery aneurysms. J Neurosurg. 2011;114(4):1154–8.

15. Lee SH, Chung Y, Ryu JW, Choi SK, Kwun BD. Surgical revascularization for the treatment of complex anterior cerebral artery aneurysms: experience and illustrative review. World Neurosurg. 2018;111:e507–18.
16. Kim LJ, Albuquerque FC, McDougall C, Spetzler RF. Combined surgical and endovascular treatment of a recurrent A3-A3 junction aneurysm unsuitable for stand-alone clip ligation or coil occlusion. Technical note. Neurosurg Focus. 2005;18(2):E6.
17. Meybodi AT, Lawton MT, Griswold D, Mokhtari P, Payman A, Yousef S, Tabani H, Benet A. Anterior temporal artery-to-anterior cerebral artery bypass: anatomic feasibility of a novel intracranial-intracranial revascularization technique. World Neurosurg. 2017;99:667–73.

Anterior Cerebral Artery-Radial Artery-Anterior Cerebral Artery Bypass

9

Jianping Song and Wei Zhu

Abstract

For a complex intracranial aneurysm originating from the A2 and beyond, in situ side-to-side bypass may be sufficient for cerebral revascularization with aneurysm trapping. Reanastomosis and reimplantation may also be considered alternative treatment modalities. However, in some specific cases with contradictions to all abovementioned bypass techniques, bypass with interposition grafts may be the last resort for treatment. A short radial artery (RA) was usually harvested as the interpositional graft.

Here, we present a case of a recurrent aneurysm in the A2 segment of the anterior cerebral artery (ACA) that was treated by ACA-RA-ACA bypass with proximal trapping.

Keywords

Anterior cerebral artery · Intracranial aneurysm · Intracranial-intracranial bypass Radial artery · Reanastomosis Revascularization

J. Song · W. Zhu (✉)
Huashan Hospital, Shanghai Medical College, Fudan University, Shanghai, China
e-mail: drzhuwei@fudan.edu.cn

9.1 Introduction

For a complex intracranial aneurysm originating from the A2 and beyond, in situ side-to-side bypass may be sufficient for cerebral revascularization with aneurysm trapping. Reanastomosis and reimplantation may also be considered alternative treatment modalities. However, in some specific cases with contradictions to all abovementioned bypass techniques, bypass with interposition grafts may be the last resort for treatment. A short radial artery (RA) was usually harvested as the interpositional graft.

Here, we present a case of a recurrent aneurysm in the A2 segment of the anterior cerebral artery (ACA) that was treated by ACA-RA-ACA bypass with proximal trapping.

9.2 Case

A 62-year-old woman was diagnosed with a fusion aneurysm in the A2 segment of the ACA 6 months prior. The aneurysm was treated with stenting at that time; however, follow-up digital subtraction angiography (DSA) showed aneurysm recurrence on both the proximal and the distal ends of the stent (Fig. 9.1). No neurological deficits were present. A side-to-side A3-A3 bypass with aneurysm trapping was first planned for this patient. However, angiography of her left internal carotid artery (ICA) showed that the left

Y. Mao et al. (eds.), *Surgical Atlas of Cerebral Revascularization*,
https://doi.org/10.1007/978-981-16-0374-7_9

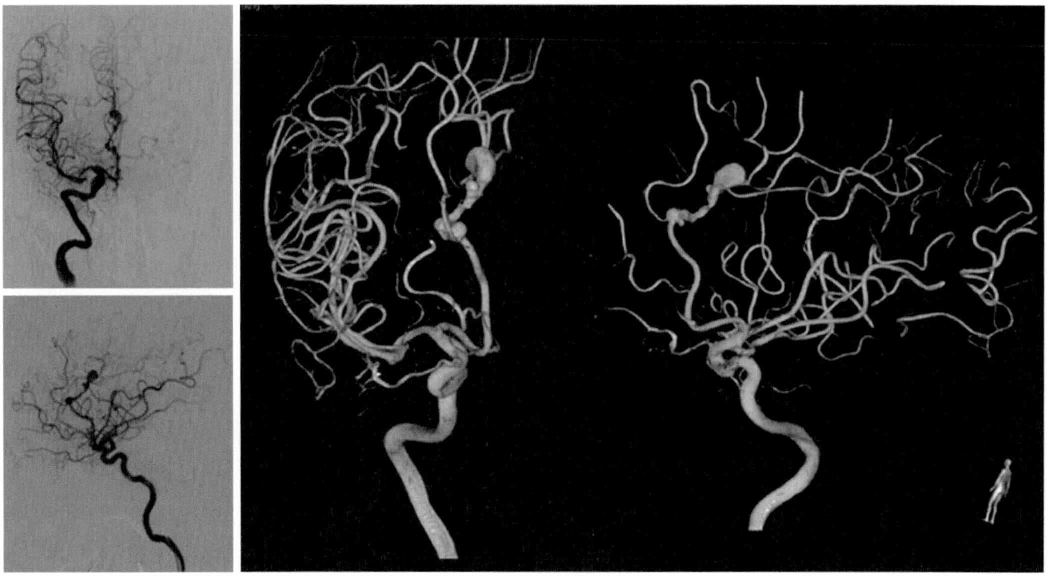

Fig. 9.1 At the 6-month follow-up, DSA (right ICA) showed aneurysm recurrence on both the proximal and the distal ends of the stent

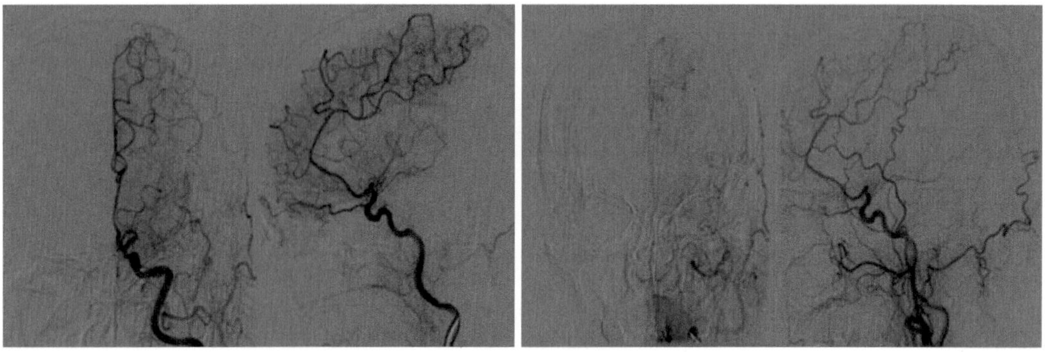

Fig. 9.2 At the 6-month follow-up, DSA (left ICA) showed that the left middle cerebral artery was occluded, and its dominating area was compensated by the left ACA

middle cerebral artery was occluded, and its dominating area was compensated by the left ACA (Fig. 9.2). Therefore, temporary occlusion of the left ACA during A3-A3 bypass would lead to a significant risk of ischemia in the left hemisphere.

Considering that A3-A3 bypass was not applicable for this patient and that end-to-end bypass after aneurysm resection is also difficult, we decided to use the RA as a short graft for proximal ACA and distal ACA bypass and then trap the aneurysm. Because the paracentral artery seemed to originate from the aneurysm body, so only proximal trapping could be achieved to allow for some backflow into this important branch (Fig. 9.3).

9.3 Details of the Procedure

During the operation, the patient was placed supine in a headholder, with the head turned 70° to the right and angled 45° upwards, allowing gravity to naturally retract the right frontal lobe for aneurysm exposure. A 6 cm × 6 cm bone window crossing the midline was made. After opening the dura and performing meticulous dissection under a microscope, the fusiform aneurysm was

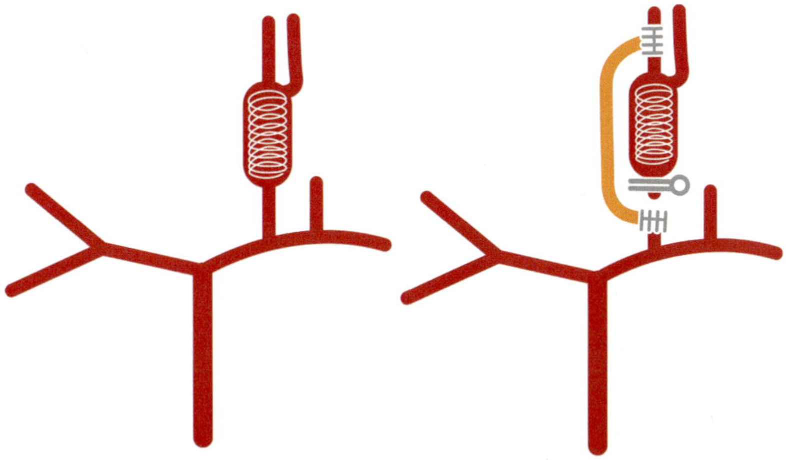

Fig. 9.3 Surgical plan: A3-RA-A3 bypass and proximal aneurysm trapping

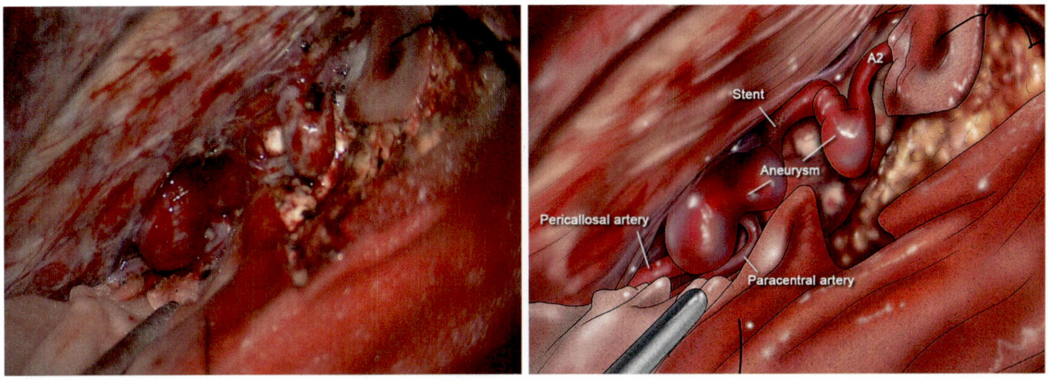

Fig. 9.4 After opening the dura and performing meticulous dissection under a microscope, the fusiform aneurysm was exposed, and a stent could be seen inside. The ACA was enlarged on each side of the stent because of the recurrent aneurysm. The paracentral artery originated from the aneurysm body

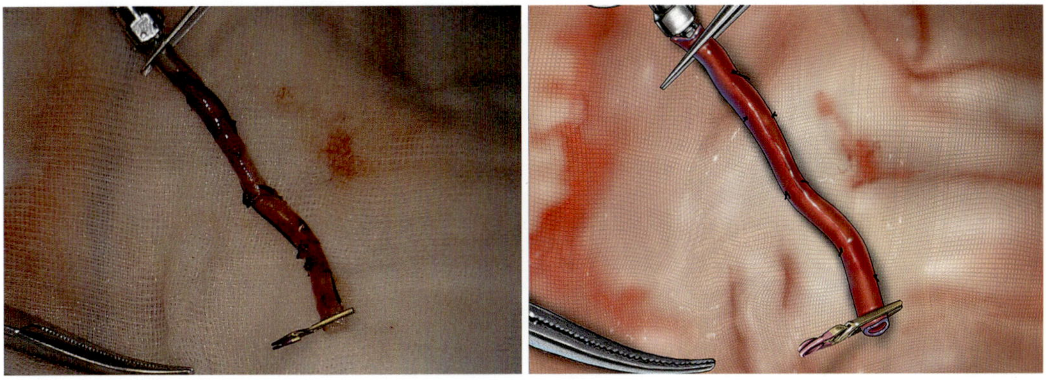

Fig. 9.5 The RA was harvested as an interpositional graft. The pressure dilation technique was used to prevent graft vasospasm

exposed, and a stent could be seen inside. The ACA was enlarged on each side of the stent because of the recurrent aneurysm. The paracentral artery originated from the aneurysm body (Fig. 9.4).

The RA was harvested as an interpositional graft. The pressure dilation technique was used to prevent graft vasospasm (Fig. 9.5).

A healthy segment of the pericallosal artery beyond the aneurysm was selected as the recipient artery and was temporarily occluded, and a rubber stripe was inserted beneath the vessel in preparation for the anastomosis (Fig. 9.6). The arteriotomy on the recipient artery was marked with methylene blue and then cut open in a linear fashion with microsurgical scissors (Fig. 9.7). The distal end of the graft was sutured to the recipient artery in an end-to-side fashion. Anchor stitches were first made on the toe and heel of the anastomosis using 9–0 Prolene sutures (Fig. 9.8).

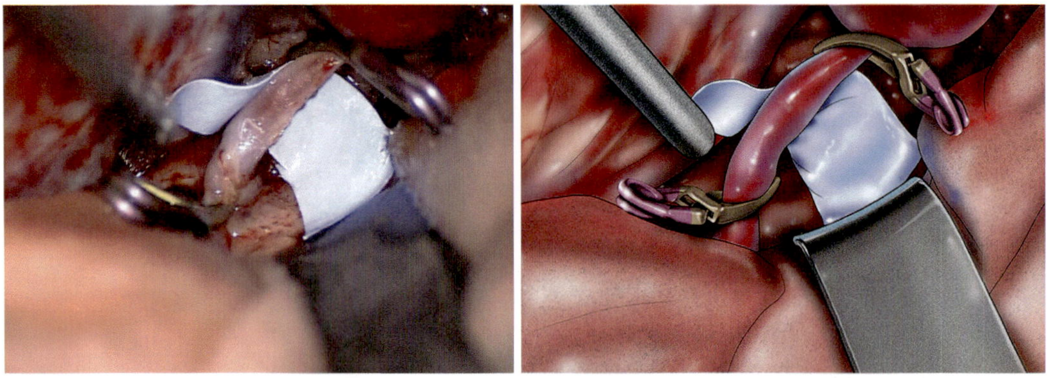

Fig. 9.6 A healthy segment of the pericallosal artery beyond the aneurysm was selected as the recipient artery and was temporarily occluded, and a rubber stripe was inserted beneath the vessel in preparation for anastomosis

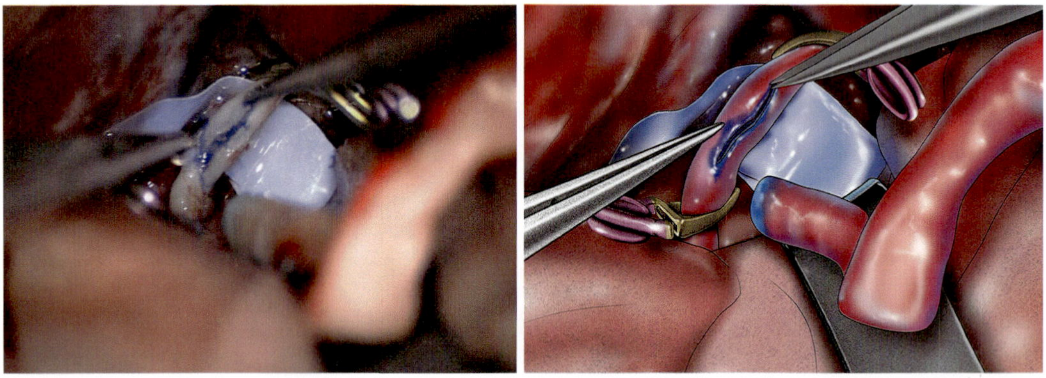

Fig. 9.7 The arteriotomy on the recipient artery was marked with methylene blue and then cut open in a linear fashion with microsurgical scissors

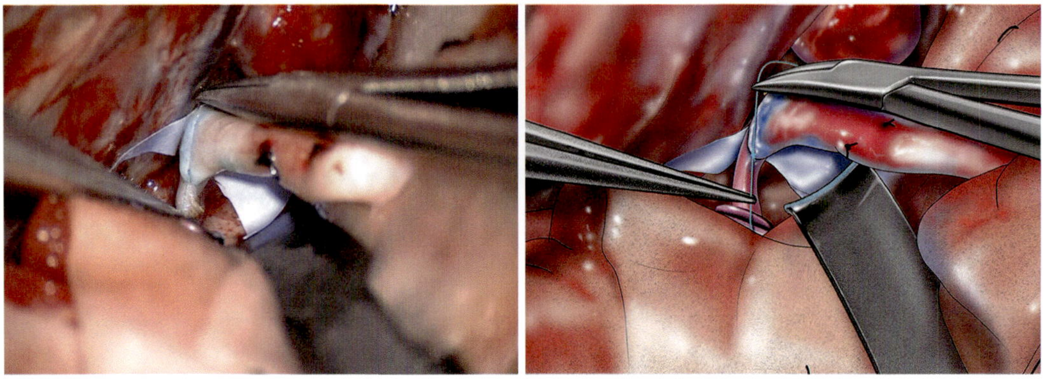

Fig. 9.8 The distal end of the graft was sutured to the recipient artery in an end-to-side fashion. Anchor stitches were first made on the toe and heel of the anastomosis using 9–0 Prolene sutures

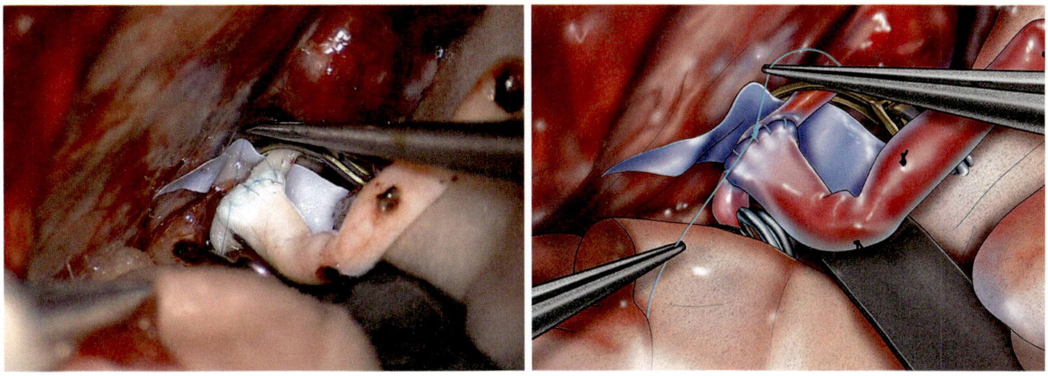

Fig. 9.9 The sidewalls of the anastomosis were sutured in an interrupted fashion. The back wall was sutured first

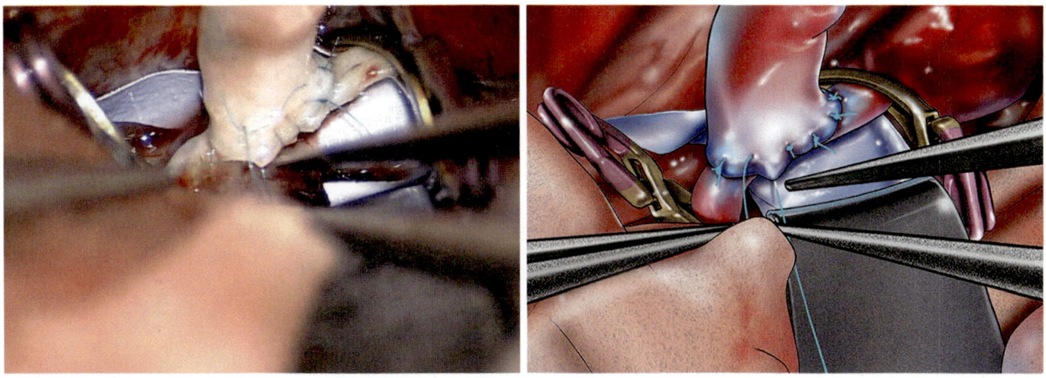

Fig. 9.10 Then, the sidewall close to the surgeon was also sutured

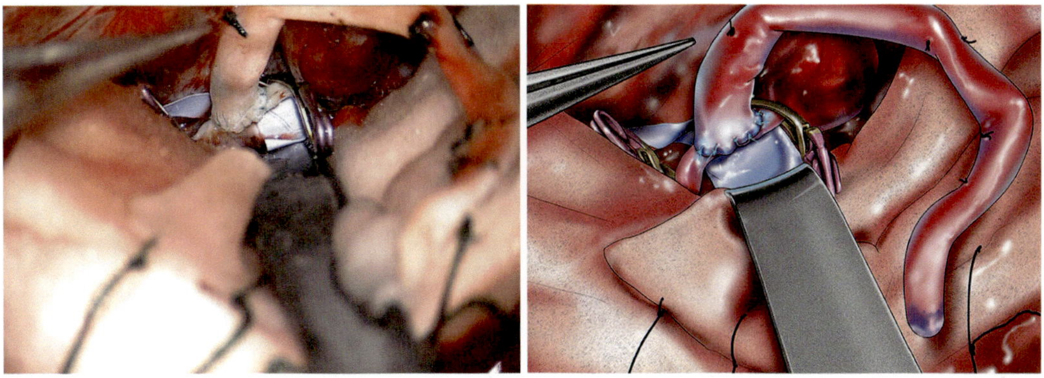

Fig. 9.11 Distal anastomosis was completed

Then, the sidewalls of the anastomosis were sutured in an interrupted fashion (Figs. 9.9 and 9.10). After distal anastomosis was accomplished (Fig. 9.11), the temporary clips were released to examine the patency of the anastomosis (Fig. 9.12), and then a temporary clip was placed on the RA graft.

Next, the A2 segment of the right ACA proximal to the aneurysm was temporarily occluded for proximal anastomosis (Fig. 9.13). This

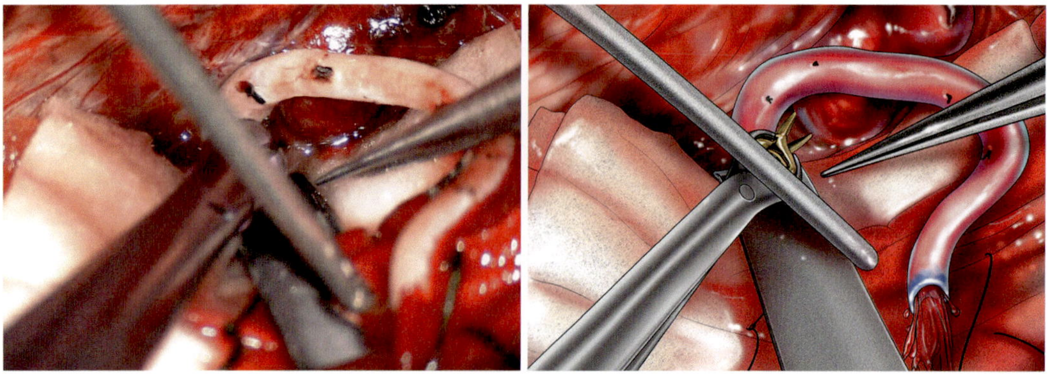

Fig. 9.12 The temporary clips were released to examine the patency of the anastomosis. Blood flushed out on the proximal end of the RA graft

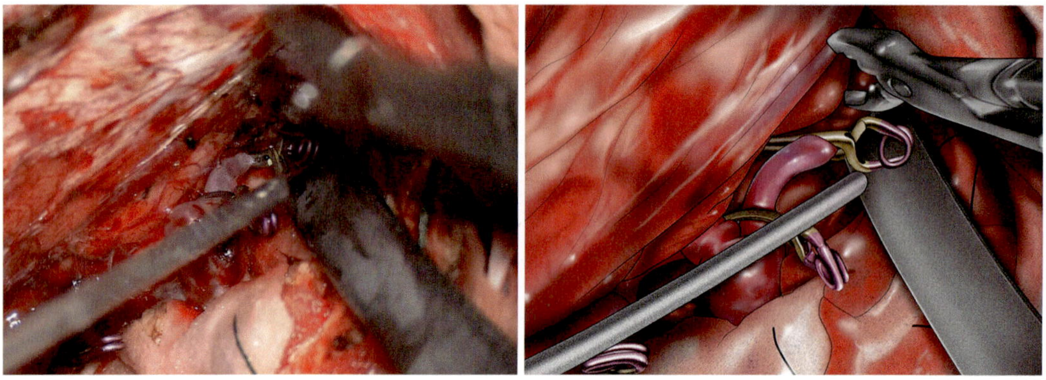

Fig. 9.13 The A2 segment of the right ACA proximal to the aneurysm was temporarily occluded for proximal anastomosis

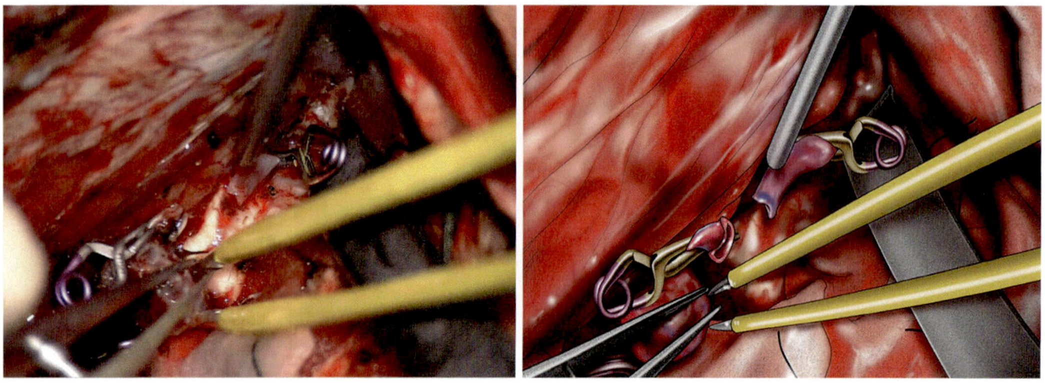

Fig. 9.14 The donor A2 segment was transected

donor A2 segment was transected and cut in a fish-mouth manner to match the caliber of the RA graft for end-to-end anastomosis. The intima edges of the stoma were marked with methylene blue (Figs. 9.14, 9.15, and 9.16), and the end-to-end anastomosis was finished with interrupted sutures. After the anastomosis, small amounts of oozing were controlled by

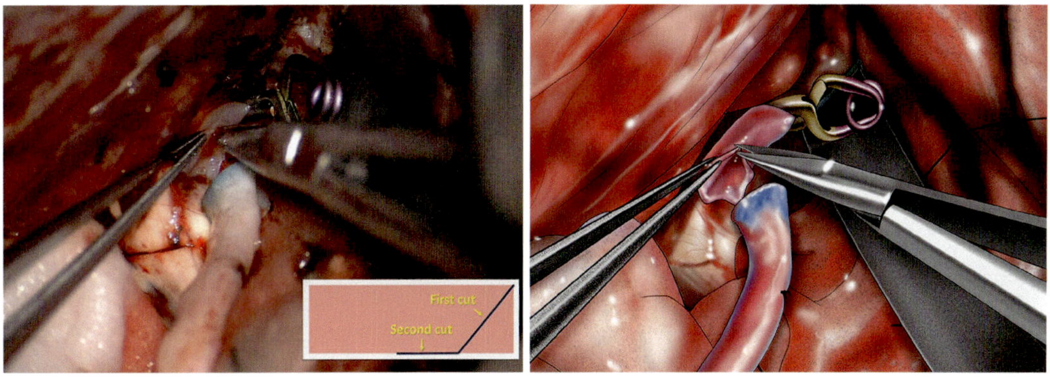

Fig. 9.15 The donor A2 segment was cut in a fish-mouth manner to match the caliber of the RA graft

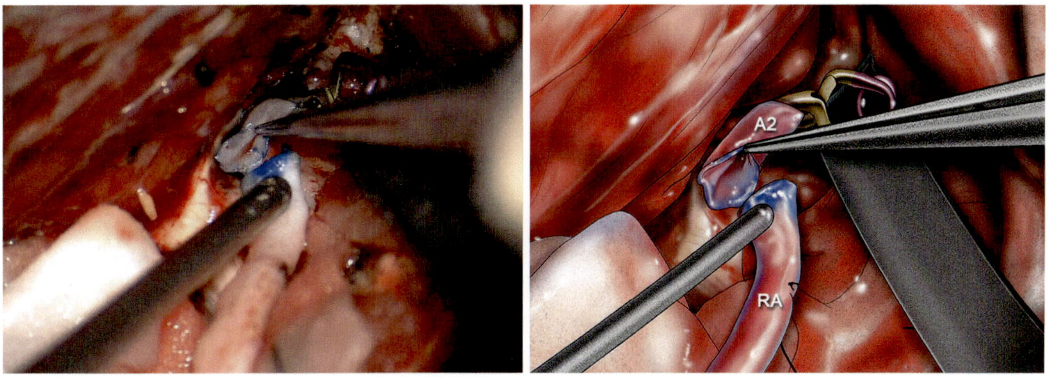

Fig. 9.16 The intima edges of the stoma were marked with methylene blue

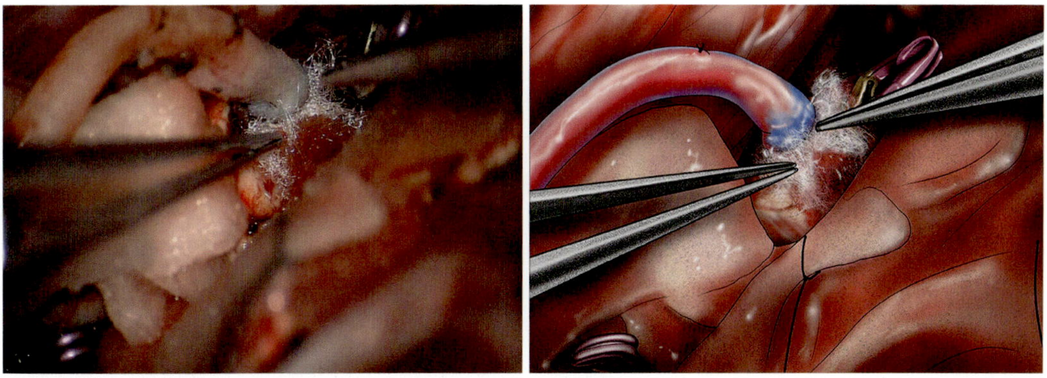

Fig. 9.17 After end-to-end anastomosis, a small amount of oozing was controlled by Surgicel

Surgicel (Fig. 9.17), and the aneurysm was proximally occluded after ACA-RA-ACA bypass (Fig. 9.18).

However, the intraoperative motor evoked potentials (MEPs) decreased gradually after the procedure. We checked the vessels with Doppler ultrasound and detected occlusion at the distal end of the RA graft; thus, the graft was cut open with a small incision, the blood clots were flushed out with heparinized saline, and the graft was closed (Fig. 9.19). The MEPs recovered very soon after clot removal.

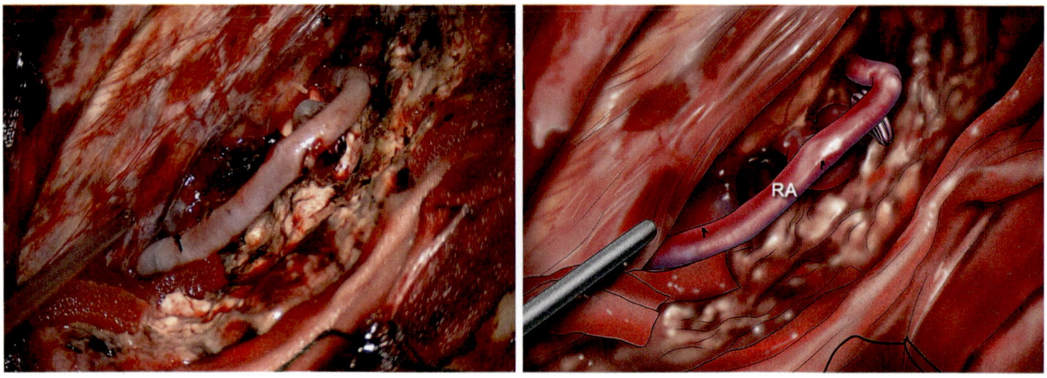

Fig. 9.18 The aneurysm was proximally occluded after ACA-RA-ACA bypass

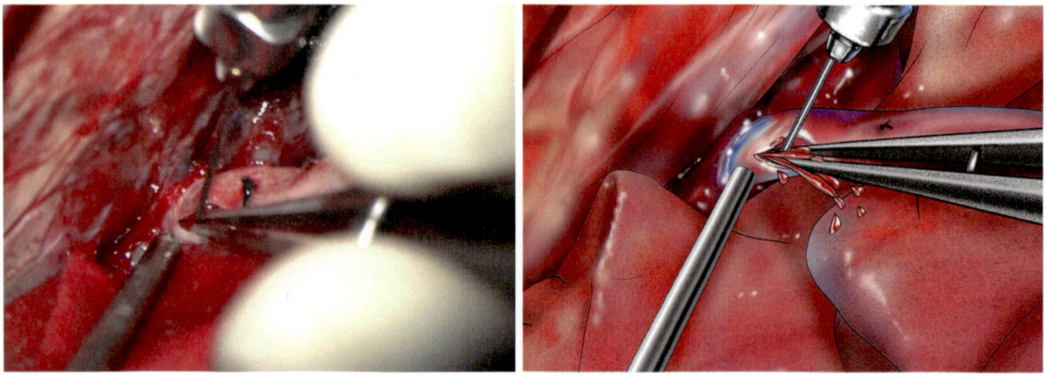

Fig. 9.19 Doppler ultrasound detected occlusion at the distal end of the RA graft. Then, the graft was cut open with a small incision, the blood clots were flushed out with heparinized saline, and the graft was closed

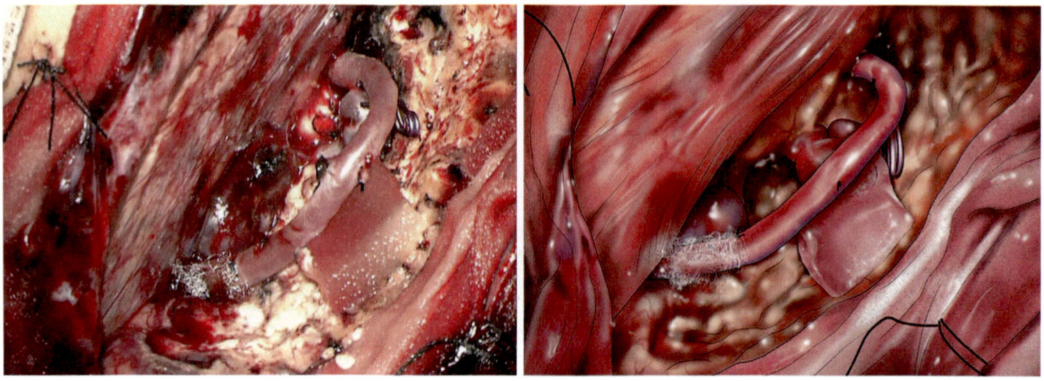

Fig. 9.20 An overview of ACA-RA-ACA bypass with proximal occlusion of the aneurysm

After ACA-RA-ACA bypass with proximal occlusion of the aneurysm (Fig. 9.20), intraoperative DSA confirmed patency of the RA graft. The proximal part of the aneurysm was not visualized, and the distal reflux blood flow preserved the patency of the right paracentral artery (red arrow) (Fig. 9.21). The patient was stable without neurological sequelae after the operation.

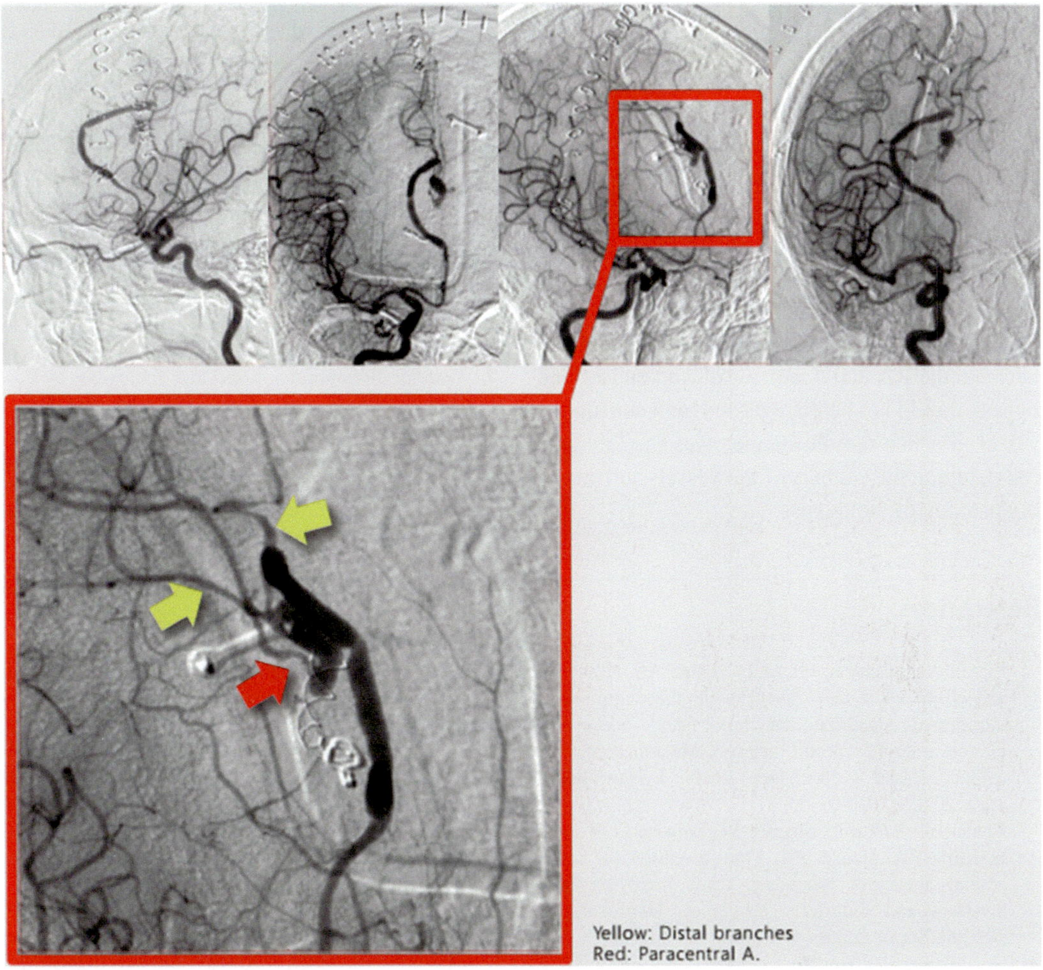

Fig. 9.21 Intraoperative DSA confirmed patency of the RA graft. The proximal part of the aneurysm was not visualized, and the distal reflux blood flow preserved the patency of the right paracentral artery (red arrow)

9.4 Comment

Is bypass outdated in the flow diverter era? Currently, the procedure to place a flow-diverting stent is relatively safe, with a very low immediate occlusion rate. However, the incidence of complete occlusion at 6 months is approximately 75–80%. The retreatment rate after placing a flow diverter is more than 10%. The periprocedural complications may be unpredictable but are fatal, and the overall complication rate is 10–15%. The overall perioperative morbidity and mortality rates range from 1% to 10%. Rerupture, delayed/non-aneurysmal intraparenchymal hemorrhage, perforator occlusion, stroke, and stent stenosis are the major complications of flow diverters. The efficacy of off-label usages of flow diverters is also contentious. Life-long anticoagulant therapy may be mandatory for some patients [1–10]. Therefore, bypass techniques are still an important skill in the arsenal of neurovascular surgeons.

In this case, aneurysm recurrence on both the proximal and distal ends of the stent obviated the possibility of endovascular retreatment. The special contradiction of left MCA occlusion with left ACA compensation weakened the tolerance of the left ACA to temporary occlusion, and side-to-side ACA-ACA bypass was too risky. The RA was harvested as a short interpositional graft for bypass, and only proximal trapping could be achieved to allow some backflow into the paracentral artery. Additionally, in this case, prolonged temporary occlusion due to two technically challenging deep bypasses raised concerns about the risk of ischemia. Therefore, end-to-side distal bypass was performed first to ensure blood perfusion into the eloquent area during the first temporary occlusion. A mismatch between the RA and donor A2 during end-to-end bypass should not be disregarded, and cutting the vessel in a fish-mouth manner was the key step for matching the calibers of the vessels and ensuring patency of the bypass.

References

1. Fiorella D, Gache L, Frame D, Arthur AS. How safe and effective are flow diverters for the treatment of unruptured small/medium intracranial aneurysms of the internal carotid artery? Meta-analysis for evidence-based performance goals. J Neurointerv Surg. 2020;12(9):869–73.
2. Chancellor B, Raz E, Shapiro M, Tanweer O, Nossek E, Riina HA, Nelson PK. Flow diversion for intracranial aneurysm treatment: trials involving flow diverters and long-term outcomes. Neurosurgery. 2020;86(Suppl 1):S36–45.
3. Gory B, Berge J, Bonafe A, Pierot L, Spelle L, Piotin M, Biondi A, Cognard C, Mounayer C, Sourour N, Barbier C, Desal H, Herbreteau D, Chabert E, Brunel H, Ricolfi F, Anxionnat R, Decullier E, Huot L, Turjman F. Flow diverters for intracranial aneurysms: the DIVERSION national prospective cohort study. Stroke. 2019;50(12):3471–80.
4. Girdhar G, Andersen A, Pangerl E, Jahanbekam R, Ubl S, Nguyen K, Wainwright J, Wolf MF. Thrombogenicity assessment of Pipeline Flex, Pipeline Shield, and FRED flow diverters in an in vitro human blood physiological flow loop model. J Biomed Mater Res A. 2018;106(12):3195–202.
5. Kiyofuji S, Graffeo CS, Perry A, Murad MH, Flemming KD, Lanzino G, Rangel-Castilla L, Brinjikji W. Meta-analysis of treatment outcomes of posterior circulation non-saccular aneurysms by flow diverters. J Neurointerv Surg. 2018;10(5):493–9.
6. Pumar JM, Mosqueira A, Cuellar H, Dieguez B, Guimaraens L, Masso J, Miralbes S, Blanco-Ulla M, Souto-Bayarri M, Vazquez-Herrero F. Expanding the use of flow diverters beyond their initial indication: treatment of small unruptured aneurysms. J Neurointerv Surg. 2018;10(3):245–8.
7. Rajah G, Narayanan S, Rangel-Castilla L. Update on flow diverters for the endovascular management of cerebral aneurysms. Neurosurg Focus. 2017;42(6):E2.
8. Griessenauer CJ, Piske RL, Baccin CE, Pereira B, Reddy AS, Thomas AJ, Abud TG, Ogilvy CS. Flow diverters for treatment of 160 ophthalmic segment aneurysms: evaluation of safety and efficacy in a multicenter cohort. Neurosurgery. 2017;80(5):726–32.
9. Brinjikji W, Murad MH, Lanzino G, Cloft HJ, Kallmes DF. Endovascular treatment of intracranial aneurysms with flow diverters: a meta-analysis. Stroke. 2013;44(2):442–7.
10. Kojima M, Irie K, Fukuda T, Arai F, Hirose Y, Negoro M. The study of flow diversion effects on aneurysm using multiple enterprise stents and two flow diverters. Asian J Neurosurg. 2012;7(4):159–65.

Carotid Endarterectomy

10

Qingzhu An and Wei Zhu

Abstract

Across the world, stroke is the second leading cause of death among people over 60 years and the second leading cause of disability among people of all ages. Extracranial carotid artery stenosis has been associated with approximately 16% of all strokes and 20% of ischemic strokes alone. Carotid endarterectomy (CEA) is a means for the secondary prevention of stroke caused by embolization from carotid plaques. Since the first description of CEA for the prevention of stroke, the operation has been widely debated and often criticized; however, the number of endarterectomy procedures performed annually has steadily increased, especially in China. Multiple major randomized controlled trials have established the benefit of CEA in stroke prevention. Altogether, four important studies (NASCET, ECST, ACAS, ACST) have proposed criteria for surgery: symptomatic patients with stenosis >50%, provided that the surgical morbidity/mortality (M/M) rate is <6%; and asymptomatic patients with stenosis >60%, provided that the M/M rate is <3%. In this chapter, we focus on the surgical techniques and procedures of CEA.

Keywords

Atherosclerotic plaque · Carotid artery
Carotid endarterectomy · Stroke · Surgery

10.1 Introduction

Across the world, stroke is the second leading cause of death among people over 60 years and the second leading cause of disability among people of all ages. Extracranial carotid artery stenosis has been associated with approximately 16% of all strokes and 20% of ischemic strokes alone. Carotid endarterectomy (CEA) is a means for the secondary prevention of stroke caused by embolization from carotid plaques. Since the first description of CEA for the prevention of stroke, the operation has been widely debated and often criticized; however, the number of endarterectomy procedures performed annually has steadily increased, especially in China. Multiple major randomized controlled trials have established the benefit of CEA in stroke prevention. Altogether, four important studies (NASCET, ECST, ACAS, ACST) have proposed criteria for surgery: symptomatic patients with stenosis >50%, provided that the surgical morbidity/mortality (M/M) rate is <6%; and asymptomatic patients with stenosis >60%, provided that the M/M rate is <3% [1–4].

Q. An · W. Zhu (✉)
Huashan Hospital, Shanghai Medical College, Fudan University, Shanghai, China
e-mail: drzhuwei@fudan.edu.cn

Y. Mao et al. (eds.), *Surgical Atlas of Cerebral Revascularization*,
https://doi.org/10.1007/978-981-16-0374-7_10

In this chapter, we focus on the surgical techniques and procedures of CEA.

10.2 Case

A 71-year-old male presented with paroxysmal weakness of the left limbs for 3 months. Physical examination before the operation showed that his Glasgow coma score was 13, and the muscle strength of all extremities was grade 5/5. Digital subtraction angiography (DSA) confirmed right internal carotid artery (ICA) stenosis (Fig. 10.1). CEA was planned for this patient (Fig. 10.2).

10.3 Details of the Procedure

During the operation, the patient was placed in the supine position, and the head was turned slightly to the contralateral side, with the neck slightly extended. The skin incision was marked along the anterior margin of the sternocleidomastoid muscle. A small L-shaped mark was drawn to indicate the angle of the mandible. Electrophysiological monitoring electrodes were connected to the scalp (Fig. 10.3).

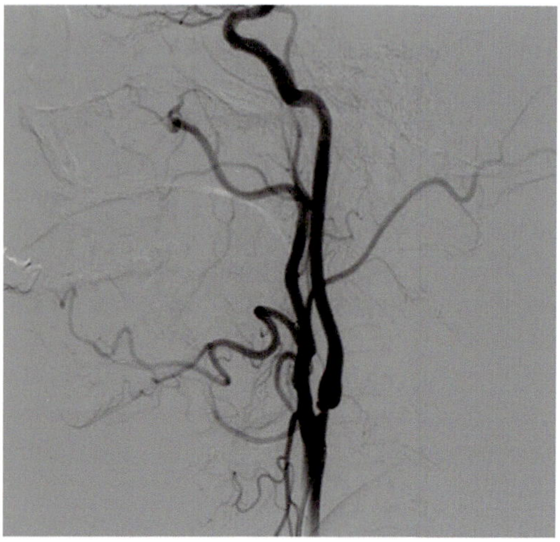

Fig. 10.1 Preoperative DSA confirmed right ICA stenosis

First, the skin and the platysma muscle were incised, while protecting the parotid fascia. The external jugular vein under the platysma muscle was doubly ligated and divided (Fig. 10.4). The dissection was carried along the anterior margin of the sternocleidomastoid muscle. Once the sternocleidomastoid muscle was free from the cervical fascia, the carotid system could be gently palpated through the fascia (Fig. 10.5). The transverse facial vein elevated by a vessel clamp was often encountered just superficial to the carotid bifurcation, serving as a reliable intraoperative anatomic landmark. This vein was doubly ligated and divided. The wound was held open with a self-retaining retractor (Fig. 10.6). The blades of the retractor were kept superficial on the medial side to avoid retraction injury to the laryngeal nerves; the retractor may, however, be placed more deeply on the lateral side.

The common, internal, and external carotid arteries (CCA, ICA, and ECA) and superior thyroid artery were all carefully isolated (Fig. 10.7). The hypoglossal nerve could be seen on the surface of the ECA. Silk tacking sutures (4–0) were applied to hold the carotid sheath open, thereby lifting the carotid bulb somewhat out of its bed and facilitating the surgical approach to the vessel.

The arteriotomy was outlined with a marking pen beginning at the CCA and proceeding distally along the ICA beyond the plaque. Infiltration of a local anesthetic with 1% lidocaine into the carotid sinus was required if bradycardia or

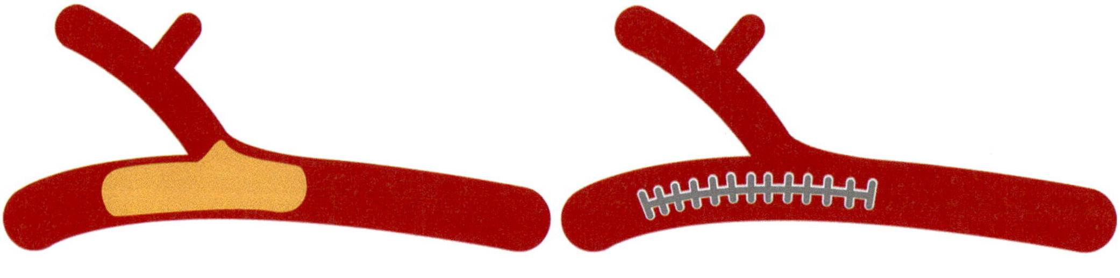

Fig. 10.2 Surgical plan: right PICA-VA reimplantation bypass combined with aneurysm trapping

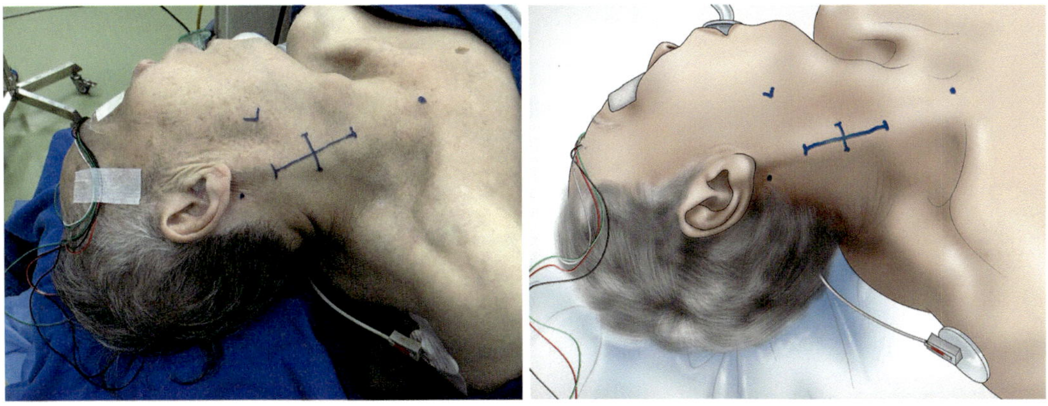

Fig. 10.3 The patient was placed in the supine position, and the head was turned slightly to the contralateral side, with the neck slightly extended. The skin incision was marked along the anterior margin of the sternocleidomastoid muscle. A small L-shaped mark was drawn to indicate the angle of the mandible. Electrophysiological monitoring electrodes were connected to the scalp

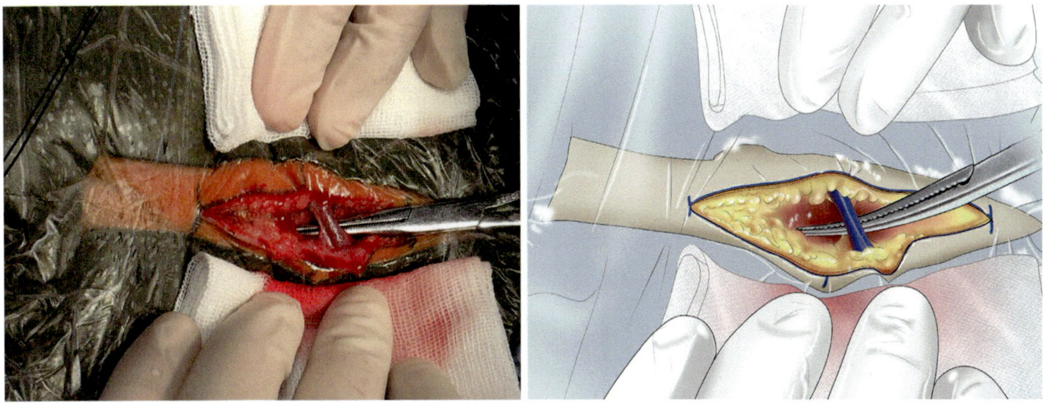

Fig. 10.4 First, the skin and the platysma muscle were incised, while protecting the parotid fascia. The external jugular vein under the platysma muscle was doubly ligated and divided

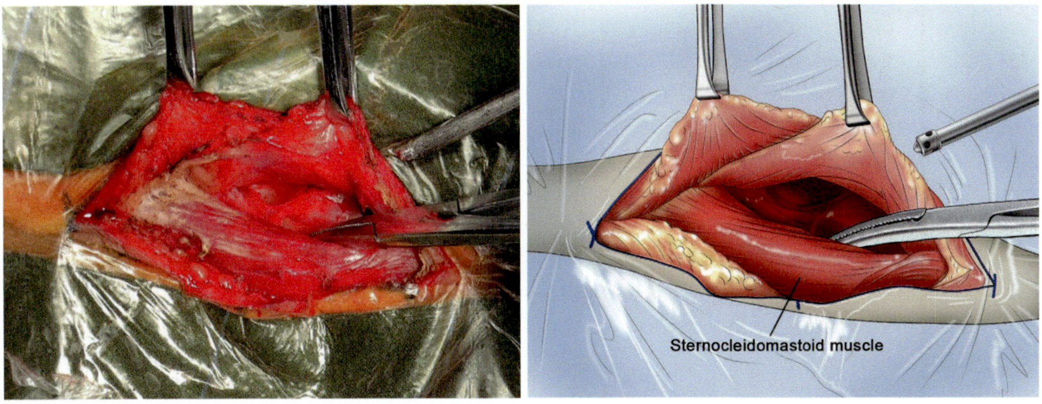

Fig. 10.5 The dissection was carried along the anterior margin of the sternocleidomastoid muscle. Once the sternocleidomastoid muscle was free from the cervical fascia, the carotid system could be gently palpated through the fascia

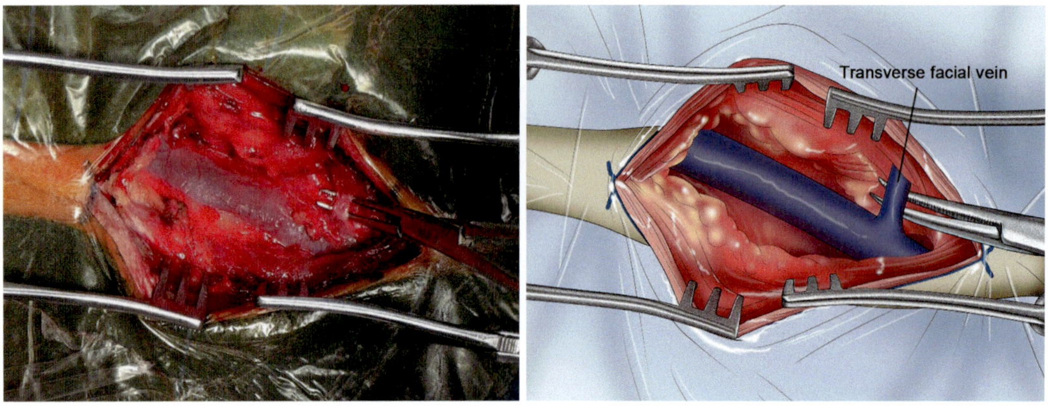

Fig. 10.6 The transverse facial vein elevated by a vessel clamp was often encountered just superficial to the carotid bifurcation, serving as a reliable intraoperative anatomic landmark. This vein was doubly ligated and divided. The wound was held open with a self-retaining retractor

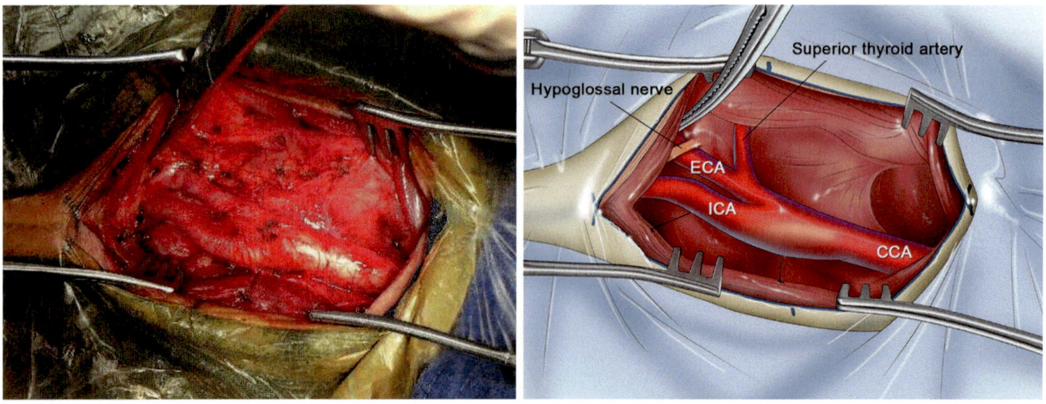

Fig. 10.7 The CCA, ICA, ECA, and superior thyroid artery were all carefully isolated

hemodynamic instability was encountered during dissection of the carotid bifurcation. The CCA was pulled downward and held with elastic rubber loops to expose more of the ICA (Fig. 10.8). The ICA was then temporarily occluded with a clamp to protect the brain from emboli detachment, and then the CCA was occluded with another clamp. The CCA and superior thyroid artery were also temporarily clipped. A fine-needle puncture on the artery wall was applied to confirm total occlusion of all relative vessels (Fig. 10.9).

After linear arteriotomy, plaque dissection was started by using a small spatula to develop a plane between the media as well as between the intima and the atherosclerotic plaque at the lateral edge of the arteriotomy. In this case, there was no natural break point proximally, and the plaque had to be cut sharply from the CCA with scissors. Then, the plaque was carefully and circumferentially dissected off the walls of the CCA, ICA, and ECA (Fig. 10.10). After the plaque was removed en bloc from the artery, the lumen was checked for any remaining plaque fragments on the wall. Any remaining plaque should be carefully removed with small ring forceps. If it was not possible to remove all remnants of the plaque at the distal end of the ICA or if the intima was loose, tacking sutures were used. These sutures were placed at the 6, 9, and

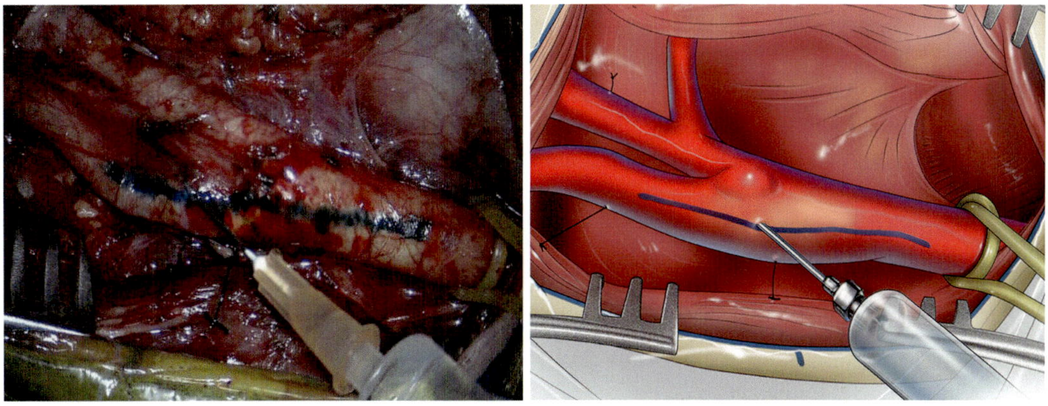

Fig. 10.8 The arteriotomy was outlined with a marking pen beginning at the CCA and proceeding distally along the ICA beyond the plaque. Infiltration of a local anesthetic with 1% lidocaine into the carotid sinus was required if bradycardia or hemodynamic instability was encountered during dissection of the carotid bifurcation. The CCA was pulled downward and held with elastic rubber loops to expose more of the ICA

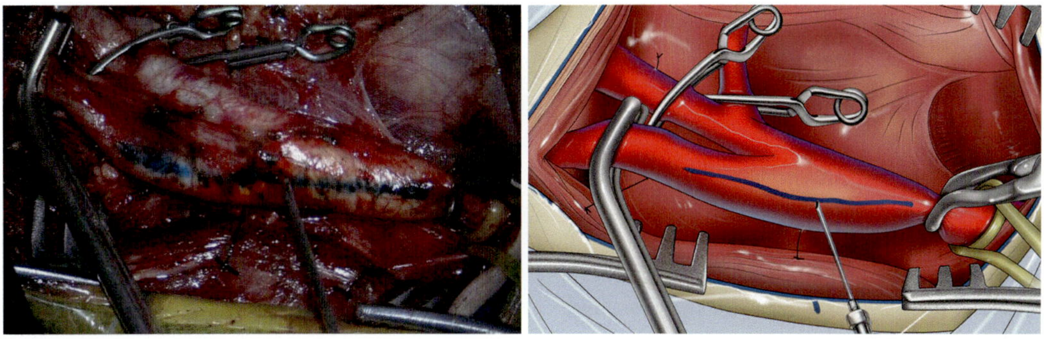

Fig. 10.9 The ICA was then temporarily occluded with a clamp to protect the brain from emboli detachment, and then the CCA was occluded with another clamp. The CCA and superior thyroid artery were also temporarily clipped. A fine-needle puncture on the artery wall was applied to confirm total occlusion of all relative vessels

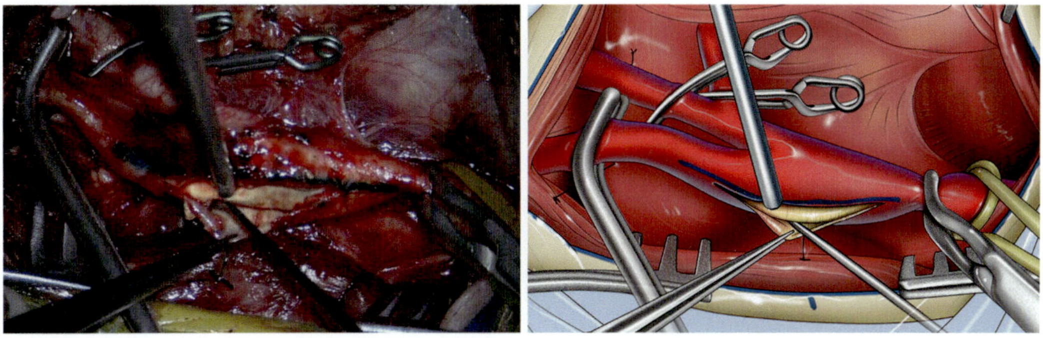

Fig. 10.10 After linear arteriotomy, plaque dissection was started by using a small spatula to develop a plane between the media as well as between the intima and the atherosclerotic plaque at the lateral edge of the arteriotomy. In this case, there was no natural break point proximally, and the plaque had to be cut sharply from the CCA with scissors. Then, the plaque was carefully and circumferentially dissected off the walls of the CCA, ICA, and ECA

12 o'clock positions, and the last suturing point was at the same site as the first stitch that started the closure, at the 3 o'clock position (Fig. 10.11).

Closure of the arteriotomy started in the distal end of the ICA. A single anchor suture was placed distal to the apex of the arteriotomy and secured with several knots. Tiny sutures were then placed in a continuous, nonlocking fashion approximately 1 mm back from the arteriotomy edge and 2 mm apart. A second suture began in the CCA where the other anchor suture was placed just proximal to the center of the arteriotomy, and sutures were also placed continuously (Fig. 10.12). When the two sutures met and could be tied together in the region of the carotid bulb, which was roughly in the middle of the arteriotomy, final closure was performed. Before tying the last stitch, the ICA was temporarily open and back-bled to ensure that no thrombosis of the ICA or inadvertent stenosis occurred due to the closure sutures. A syringe with heparinized saline and a long blunt needle was introduced into the arterial lumen between the two sutures. The lumen was then filled with heparinized saline to ensure that all air and debris were flushed out of the artery, and then the last stitch was tied (Fig. 10.13).

Final restoration of the blood flow was carried out by first releasing the ECA and CCA in sequence. This maneuver could allow for the

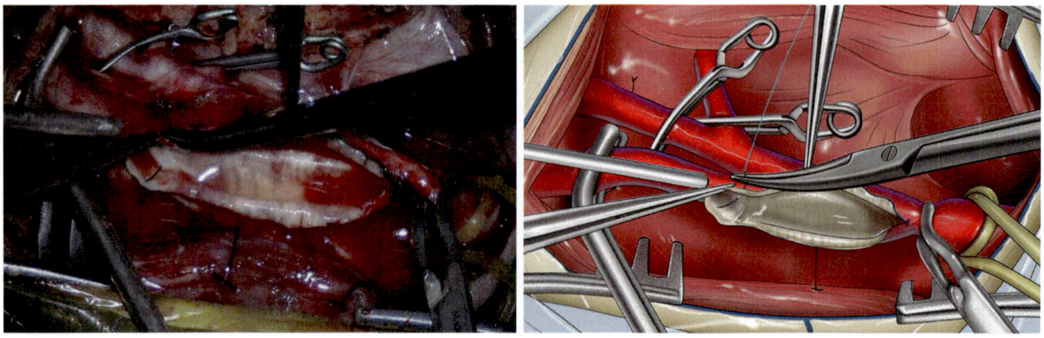

Fig. 10.11 After the plaque was removed en bloc from the artery, the lumen was checked for any remaining plaque fragments on the wall. Any remaining plaque was carefully removed with small ring forceps. If it was not possible to remove all remnants of the plaque in the distal end of the ICA or if the intima was loose, tacking sutures were used. These sutures were placed at the 6, 9, and 12 o'clock positions, and the last suture was placed at the same site as the first stitch that started the closure, at the 3 o'clock position

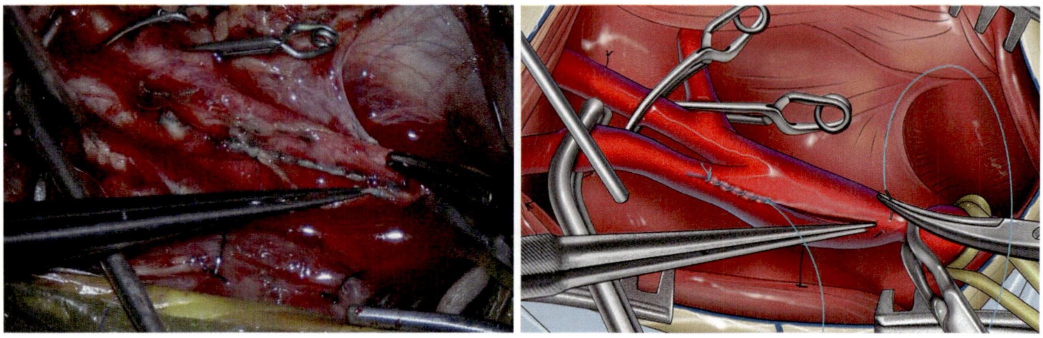

Fig. 10.12 Closure of the arteriotomy started in the distal end of the ICA. A single anchor suture was placed distal to the apex of the arteriotomy and secured with several knots. Tiny sutures were then placed in a continuous, nonlocking fashion approximately 1 mm away from the arteriotomy edge and 2 mm apart. A second suture began in the CCA where the other anchor suture was placed just proximal to the center of the arteriotomy, and the sutures were also placed continuously

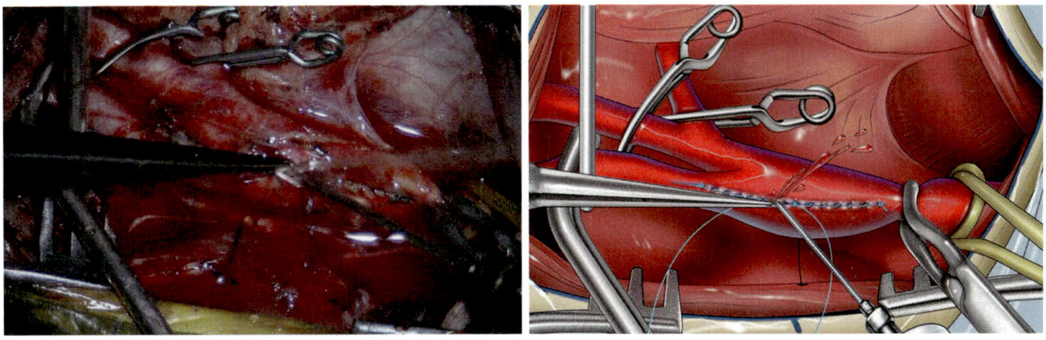

Fig. 10.13 When the two sutures met and could be tied together in the region of the carotid bulb, which was roughly the middle of the arteriotomy, final closure was performed. Before tying the last stitch, the ICA was temporarily open and back-bled to ensure that no thrombosis of the ICA or inadvertent stenosis occurred due to the closure sutures. A syringe with heparinized saline and a long blunt needle was introduced into the arterial lumen between the two sutures. The lumen was then filled with heparinized saline to ensure that all air and debris were flushed out of the artery before the last stitch was tied

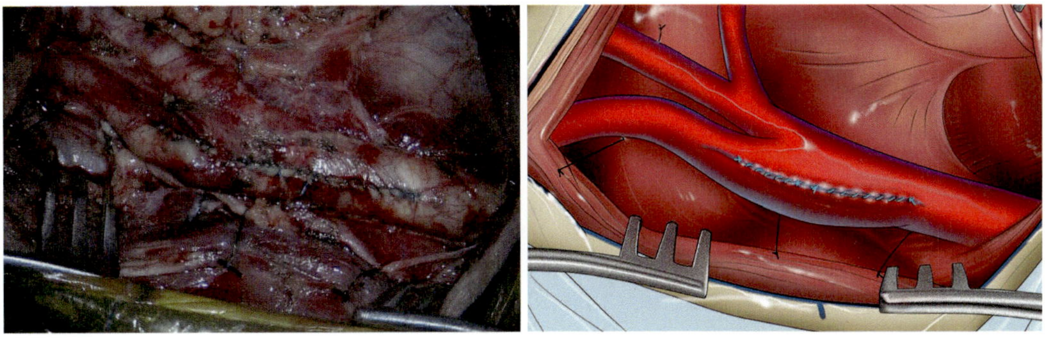

Fig. 10.14 Final restoration of the blood flow was carried out by first releasing the ECA and CCA in sequence. This maneuver could allow for the potentially remaining debris to be flushed into the ECA. Then, the clamps on the ICA were removed to restore cerebral circulation. With a meticulous closure, there was little need for additional hemostatic agents

potentially remaining debris to be flushed into the ECA. Then, the clamps on the ICA were removed to restore cerebral circulation. With meticulous closure, there was little need for additional hemostatic agents (Fig. 10.14).

The follow-up DSA one year later demonstrated patency of the right ICA without stenosis (Fig. 10.15).

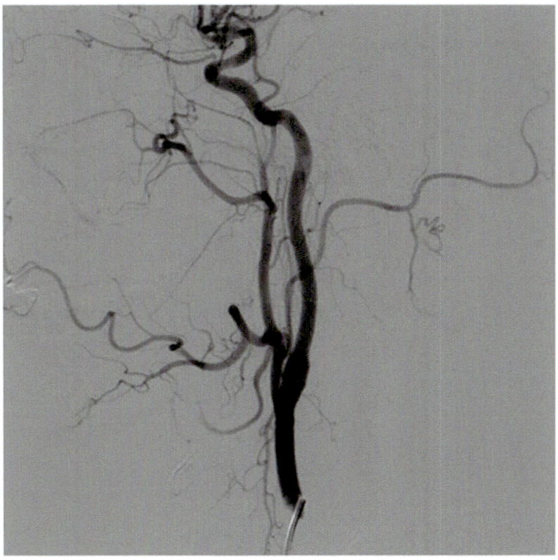

Fig. 10.15 The follow-up DSA one year later demonstrated patency of the right ICA without stenosis

10.4 Comment

In the treatment of extracranial carotid disease, the most difficult aspect is deciding who will benefit from CEA. Despite the emergence of and advances in carotid angioplasty and stenting, CEA should remain the first-line intervention for the right group of patients. CEA should be performed only at institutions with a high volume of patients and a proven low M/M rate. Although there are numerous ways to perform CEA, several basic principles of carotid reconstruction must always be applied. We prefer general anesthesia with full-channel electroencephalography (EEG) and concurrent somatosensory evoked potential (SEP) monitoring, and we performed selective shunting based on the monitoring criteria. We only placed tacking sutures in a few cases due to the use of fine scissors that could trim the plaque cleanly from the ICA as it was removed. The techniques described in this chapter are in no way meant to be thought of as a "standard" method. However, after surgery, the risk of stroke is not completely eliminated because only a tiny part of the vasculature is treated and the overall underlying process (atherosclerosis) remains unchanged. Thus, there is a need for lifelong medical treatment and regular examinations.

References

1. Barnett HJ, Taylor DW, Eliasziw M, Fox AJ, Ferguson GG, Haynes RB, Rankin RN, Clagett GP, Hachinski VC, Sackett DL, Thorpe KE, Meldrum HE, Spence JD. Benefit of carotid endarterectomy in patients with symptomatic moderate or severe stenosis. North American Symptomatic Carotid Endarterectomy Trial Collaborators. N Engl J Med. 1998;339(20):1415–25.
2. Randomised trial of endarterectomy for recently symptomatic carotid stenosis: final results of the MRC European Carotid Surgery Trial (ECST). Lancet. 1998;351(9113):1379–87.
3. Endarterectomy for asymptomatic carotid artery stenosis. Executive Committee for the Asymptomatic Carotid Atherosclerosis Study. JAMA. 1995;273(18):1421–8.
4. Halliday A, Harrison M, Hayter E, Kong X, Mansfield A, Marro J, Pan H, Peto R, Potter J, Rahimi K, Rau A, Robertson S, Streifler J, Thomas D. 10-year stroke prevention after successful carotid endarterectomy for asymptomatic stenosis (ACST-1): a multicentre randomised trial. Lancet. 2010;376(9746):1074–84.

11 Computational Fluid Dynamics Study of Cerebral Revascularization for Moyamoya Disease

Fengping Zhu, Yi Qian, and Ying Mao

Abstract

Computational fluid dynamics (CFD) is a mechanical engineering branch for analyzing fluid flow, heat transfer, and associated phenomena using computer-based simulations. When the bypass for Moyamoya disease (MMD) is done, cerebral vessel remodeling starts. Such autoremodeling occurs in the first few weeks and even months after surgery and may impact the final outcome. The deployment of CFD technology in MMD has been attempted recently, as these hemodynamic parameters have been suggested to help clinicians unravel the disease pathogenesis and plan surgical intervention in MMD patients. Our group evaluated the characteristic vessel remodeling for both bypass and the internal carotid artery in MMD using CFD.

Keywords

Computational fluid dynamics · Extracranial-intracranial bypass · Moyamoya disease Pressure drop index · Revascularization · Wall shear stress

11.1 Preface

Computational fluid dynamics (CFD) is a mechanical engineering branch for analyzing fluid flow, heat transfer, and associated phenomena using computer-based simulations [1]. With advances in imaging and computer technology, CFD has been widely adopted in biomedical engineering. CFD technology can aid in calculating hemodynamic parameters in addition to flow velocities, such as total and relative pressure, wall shear, and volume flow. In cerebrovascular disease, CFD is usually used to characterize the hemodynamic features of the formation, growth, and rupture of aneurysms [2–6]. Besides, CFD has also been used to simulate stent implantation for intracranial stenosis [7]. Amin-Hanjani et al. applied CFD in the treatment of cerebral arteriovenous malformation (AVM), demonstrating that the wall shear stress (WSS) is high in cerebral AVM arterial feeders, which might result from high blood flows and insufficient compensation with feeder enlargement. The decreases in WSS might be regarded as a potential biomechanical factor for efficient AVM treatment [8].

11.2 Introduction: CFD Use in Moyamoya Disease

In Moyamoya disease (MMD), cerebral vessel remodeling starts when the bypass is established. Such autoremodeling occurs in the first few

F. Zhu · Y. Mao (✉)
Huashan Hospital, Shanghai Medical College, Fudan University, Shanghai, China
e-mail: maoying@fudan.edu.cn

Y. Qian
Macquarie University, Sydney, Australia

Y. Mao et al. (eds.), *Surgical Atlas of Cerebral Revascularization*,
https://doi.org/10.1007/978-981-16-0374-7_11

weeks and even months after surgery and may impact the final outcome. The deployment of CFD technology in MMD has been attempted recently, as these hemodynamic parameters have been suggested to help clinicians unravel the disease pathogenesis and plan surgical intervention in MMD patients. A few studies are investigating the hemodynamic characteristics of MMD. Seol et al. used 2D geometrical CFD models of the distal internal carotid artery (ICA) and posterior cerebral artery (PCA) to study the hemodynamics in the circle of Willis (CoW). The results demonstrated that WSS in the ICA region was relatively low. The predisposing area of MMD might be related to the distribution of shear stress. A continuous low WSS level might promote cerebral vascular smooth muscle cells' migration and cause MMD progression [9]. Charbel et al. used a computerized model to analyze the flow distribution in one case of MMD and simulate cerebral blood flow following various treatment options to decide on the optimal treatment option [10]. Kim et al. investigated the morphology and hemodynamic characteristics of MMD using the CFD technique. The MMD ICA's vascular length and tortuosity were significantly shorter and lessened than normal ICA, showing smaller curvature angles in the intracavernous and petrous segments. Higher WSS and faster blood flow in the ICA bifurcation were confirmed [11]. Our group evaluated the characteristic vessel remodeling in MMD using CFD for both bypass and the ICA [11–15].

11.3 Details of the Procedure

11.3.1 Vessel Geometry Reconstruction

Patient-specific vessel models were acquired. Images were obtained from magnetic resonance angiography (MRA). Based on the images, a commercial software package—MIMICS (Materialise' Interactive Medical Image Control System, Belgium)—was used to reconstruct and segment the vessels' 3D geometries and then generate domains for CFD simulation. Instead of using "global smoothing," manual "local smoothing" was used to preserve the 3D geometry as realistically as possible. The reconstructed geometries were then exported into ICEM CFDR (Ansys Inc., Canonsburg, PA, USA) for mesh generation.

11.3.2 CFD Modeling

The two-dimensional contours of the ICA, superficial temporal artery (STA), and CoW (left and right ICA and basilar artery (BA)) were generated from grayscale pixels. By subsequent interpolation in a normal direction, these vessels' 3D geometry was reconstructed using the contours and preventing surface noise intrusion. Surface smoothing was set to a minimum level and a few localized areas to reduce distortion and maintain the surface roughness like the actual vessel surface. Navier-Stokes equations for 3D flow with rigid walls were solved using ANSYS CFX 14 (Ansys Inc., Canonsburg, PA, USA) under steady-state flow conditions. Steady-state simulations have been proven to achieve similar time-averaged results for pulsatile calculations over a cardiac cycle [16]. The pre- and postoperative inflow boundary conditions were measured using transcranial doppler ultrasound (TCD) and/or quantitative MRA individually. Blood flow was assumed as a laminar Newtonian flow. The blood flow's dynamic viscosity and density were set as 0.0032 Pa s and 1050 kg/m^3, respectively.

The vessel outlet was extruded distally in a downstream direction to 100 mesh layers to mimic venous capacitance and allow for sufficient blood pressure recovery. Patient-specific inlet boundaries were set based on flow measurements, and zero pressure conditions were applied at all outlets. Fully developed velocity profiles mimicking the measured flow rates were obtained at the proximal inlet boundary layer, and for this reason, the domains were extruded in the upstream direction to 100 mesh layers. The total elements number ranged between 1,000,000 and 1,400,000. The inlet/outlet interfaces' grid size was fixed at 0.01 mm. The rest of the computational domain had a maximum grid size of 0.02 mm.

11.3.3 Postprocessing

WSS, flow, and pressure distribution in the arterial wall were analyzed in contour plots. To better estimate the remodeling characteristics of MMD, different hemodynamic parameters were defined and evaluated based on CFD simulations in different sections of this study.

11.4 Findings

11.4.1 The Vessel Remodeling Hemodynamic Analysis in STA-MCA Bypass

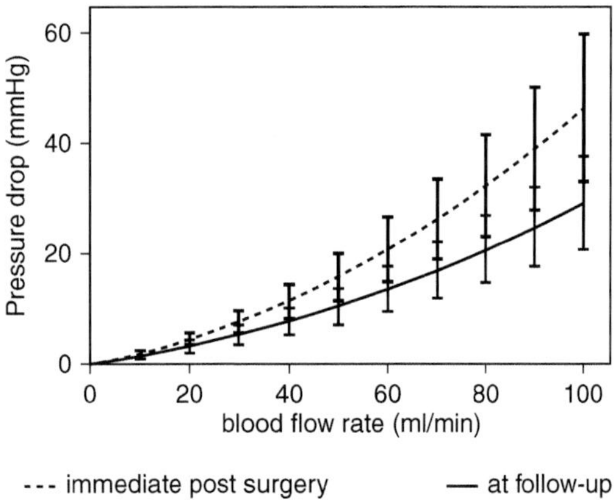

Fig. 11.1 Mean flow resistance changes due to vessel remodeling. The mean flow resistance at follow-up was decreased compared with that immediately postsurgery. This is consistent with the expansion of the bypass diameter (Reproduced from Zhu FP, Zhang Y, Higurashi M, Xu B, Gu YX, Mao Y, Morgan MK, Qian Y. Hemodynamic analysis of vessel remodelling in STA-MCA bypass for Moyamoya disease and its impact on bypass patency. J Biomech. 2014; 47(8): 1800–05)

During the late follow-up stages, the occlusion of a thriving STA-middle cerebral artery (STA-MCA) bypass with immediate excellent bypass flow may still occur. This phenomenon may be related to some patient factors, but vessel autoremodeling may also play an important role. The bypass vessels' average diameter increased from 1.35 ± 0.47 mm at the surgery to 1.60 ± 0.36 mm at follow-up. To further understand the STA-MCA bypass remodeling effect, we studied the hemodynamics of STA-MCA bypasses, measured its flow resistance coefficients, and evaluated the modifications to bypass patency over 6 months. In most cases, the flow resistance during bypass lowered (Fig. 11.1). Furthermore, the amplitude of low-frequency fluctuations (ALFFs) patterns of many brain regions were found to change with progressive cognitive decline. Notably, the most significant differences in ALFFs were observed in regions such as the prefrontal cortex (PFC), anterior cingulate cortex (ACC), and right supplemental motor area (SMA). Then, we found that the right middle frontal gyrus (MFG), right SMA, bilateral ACC, and orbitofrontal gyrus (OFG) showed the most significant correlation with Mini-Mental State Examination (MMSE) scores. Furthermore, a positive correlation with MMSE scores was found in the bilateral superior parietal lobe, inferior parietal lobe (IPL), and left caudate nucleus, while a negative correlation was found in the bilateral precuneus (PCu) (Fig. 11.1).

Our study illustrates that the WSS immediately following surgery tended to be high. This phenomenon is due to an acute change in the STA's vascular environment after the bypass. The WSS decreased as autoremodeling occurred over time (Fig. 11.2). For most STA-MCA bypasses with successful bypass, vessel autoremodeling decreased the stenosis degree of the recipient artery immediately after surgery and increased its internal diameter's uniformity over time. Therefore, the bypass's flow resistance was reduced, resulting in a higher flow rate and increasingly uniform WSS. Figure 11.3a shows that the WSS in successful cases tends to be uniform due to remodeling.

Our study also highlights the significance of the initial bypass morphology in the autoremodeling process. The WSS and flow resistance increased in the unsuccessful cases (for the cases of potentially occluded bypass, but without any abnormal symptoms) at follow-up (Fig. 11.3b). We speculate that the reason for this unexpected remodeling is most likely the significant curvature degree of STA at the time of STA-MCA bypass surgery. The bypass's initial morphology may affect the vessel's flow distribution, further resulting in different vessel remodeling patterns. If the STA trunk possesses a significant curvature, worsened autoremodeling can be expected due to the pre-existing curvature, leading to high flow resistance and potentially vessel occlusion. Therefore, to ensure the STA-MCA bypass's patency at follow-up, both the curvature of STA and the appropriate placement of the bypass vessel must be carefully considered.

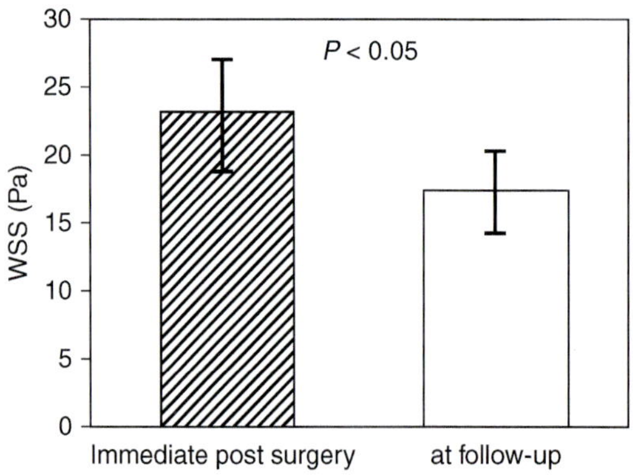

Fig. 11.2 Mean WSS change due to vessel remodeling. The mean WSS at follow-up was decreased compared with that immediately postsurgery. The decrease in WSS confirmed that vessel remodeling reduces the impedance of the bypass (Reproduced from Zhu FP, Zhang Y, Higurashi M, Xu B, Gu YX, Mao Y, Morgan MK, Qian Y. Haemodynamic analysis of vessel remodelling in STA-MCA bypass for Moyamoya disease and its impact on bypass patency. J Biomech. 2014; 47(8): 1800–05)

11.4.2 The Vessel Remodeling Hemodynamic Analysis in the ICA

Bypass surgery might help decrease the recurrent bleeding rate in the hemorrhagic type of MMD. The angiographic diminishment of Moyamoya vessels was reported after EC-IC bypass surgery due to decreased hemodynamic stress to the pathological vessels. Using CFD technology, we managed to estimate the hemodynamic modification to the ICA after bypass surgery. This study might help to understand the influence of hemodynamic changes on the outcomes of revascularization surgery. The treatment outcome was classified according to the proportion of the MCA distribution network sup-

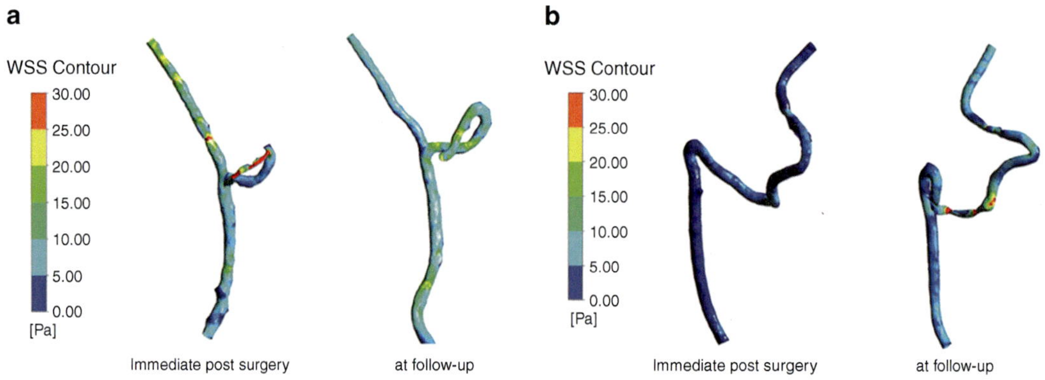

Fig. 11.3 WSS distribution in the illustrative cases due to vessel remodeling. (**a**) For the successful case, because the stenosis was resolved, the blood flowed more smoothly at follow-up, which led to a uniform WSS distribution. (**b**) For the unsuccessful case, as the bypass diameter shrank, WSS increased at follow-up (Reproduced from Zhu FP, Zhang Y, Higurashi M, Xu B, Gu YX, Mao Y, Morgan MK, Qian Y. Haemodynamic analysis of vessel remodelling in STA-MCA bypass for Moyamoya disease and its impact on bypass patency. J Biomech. 2014; 47(8): 1800–05)

plied by revascularization surgery [17]: A, more than two-thirds of the MCA distribution; B, between one-third and two-thirds of the MCA distribution; and C, less than one-third of the MCA distribution.

The pressure drop index (PDI) was defined as the difference in pressure reduction along the ICA between preoperative and follow-up status stages. The PDI can be calculated using the following formula (Formula 1):

$$\begin{aligned} \mathrm{PDI} &= \Delta P_f - \Delta P_p \\ &= \left[\left(P_{if} - P_{of}\right) - \left(P_{ip} - P_{op}\right)\right] \end{aligned} \quad (11.1)$$

where ΔP_f and ΔP_p are the calculated pressure reductions at follow-up and preoperative stages, respectively; P_{if} and P_{of} are the follow-up pressure values calculated at the inlet (proximal) and outlet (distal) sections, respectively; and P_{ip} and P_{op} are the preoperative pressure values calculated at the ICA inlet and outlet, respectively, as shown in Fig. 11.4. All units are in mmHg. We measured the pressure values at the same inlet and outlet planes in the preoperative and follow-up models [17].

The volume flow rate of the surgically treated ICA significantly decreased from 157.77 ± 50.14 ml/min to 131.28 ± 51.78 ml/min ($P < 0.01$) at follow-up (Fig. 11.5). In group A, due to the good ICA autoremodeling (e.g., stenosis progression in the terminal ICA, reduction in diameter), the flow rate in the surgically treated ICA decreased by 24.2%. While in groups B and C, the blood flow decreased by 10.5% and 3.7%, respectively [17].

The average PDIs of surgically treated ICA and nonsurgically treated ICA among all cases were −1.00 and 0.51, respectively. The PDI change in the treated ICAs was significantly different from that in the nontreated ICAs ($P < 0.01$) (Fig. 11.6).

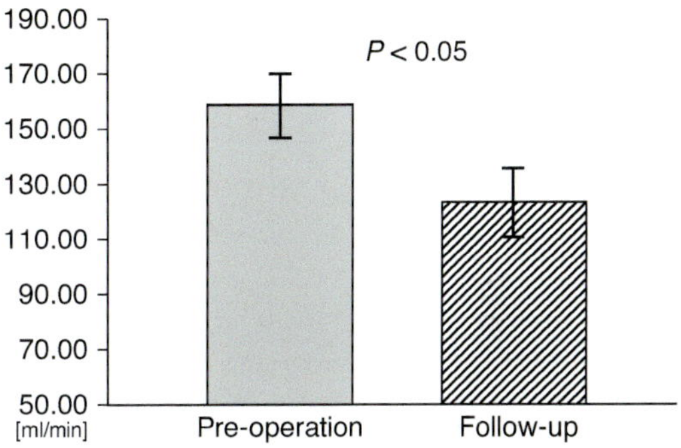

Fig. 11.5 Volume flow rate of the treated ICA preoperatively and at follow-up (Reproduced from Zhu F, Karunanithi K, Qian Y, Mao Y, Xu B, Gu Y, Zhu W, Chen L, Wang Y, Pan H, Liao Y, Morgan M. Assessing surgical treatment outcome following superficial temporal artery to middle cerebral artery bypass based on computational haemodynamic analysis. J Biomech. 2015; 48(15): 4053–58)

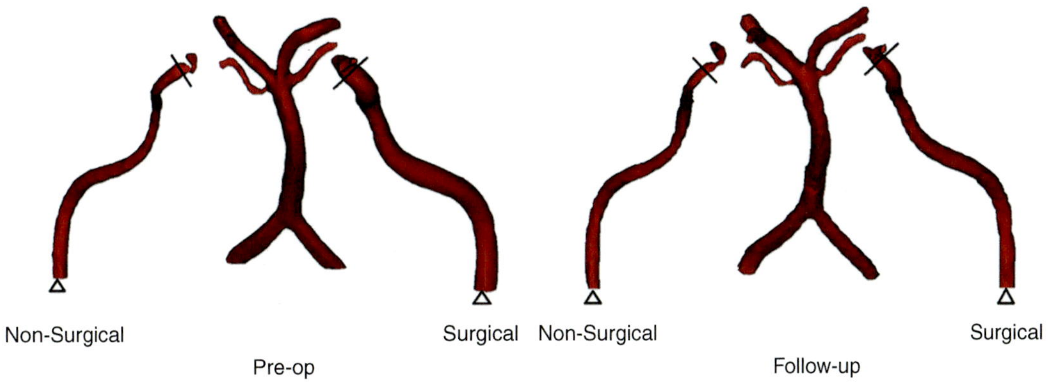

Fig. 11.4 Illustration of the planes for measuring pressure in the preoperative and follow-up CFD models. The inlet measurement plane is marked with a triangle, and the outlet measurement plane is labeled using a black line (Reproduced from Zhu F, Karunanithi K, Qian Y, Mao Y, Xu B, Gu Y, Zhu W, Chen L, Wang Y, Pan H, Liao Y, Morgan M. Assessing surgical treatment outcome following superficial temporal artery to middle cerebral artery bypass based on computational haemodynamic analysis. J Biomech. 2015; 48(15): 4053–58)

By observing the surgically treated ICA's structural and hemodynamic changes, we found that its tortuosity and diameter decreased. However, the WSS did not change (illustrated by one case in group A, Fig. 11.7).

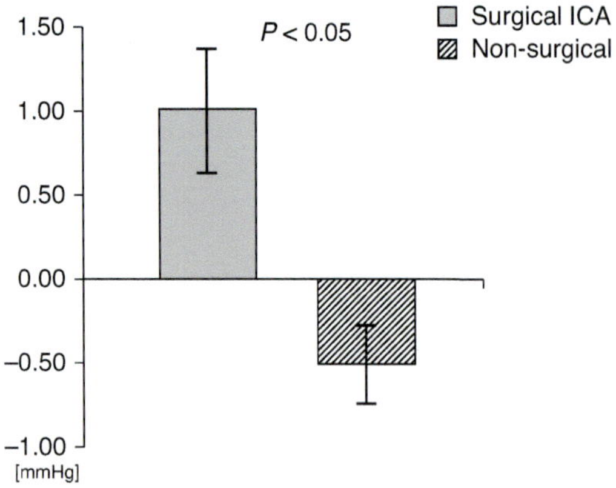

Fig. 11.6 PDIs of surgically treated and nonsurgically treated ICAs (Reproduced from Zhu F, Karunanithi K, Qian Y, Mao Y, Xu B, Gu Y, Zhu W, Chen L, Wang Y, Pan H, Liao Y, Morgan M. Assessing surgical treatment outcome following superficial temporal artery to middle cerebral artery bypass based on computational haemodynamic analysis. J Biomech. 2015; 48(15): 4053–58)

Following the observation of preoperative and follow-up ICA changes among the cases in group C, we found that the ICA diameter did not change. However, there was new and severe stenosis in the ICA trunk. The WSS at the stenotic and terminal portions of the ICA were quite different. One typical case of group C was illustrated in Fig. 11.8.

Thus, the ICA undergoes characteristic vessel remodeling after combined direct and indirect revascularization surgery, usually with decreased pressure drop and volume flow rate. Detailed CFD analysis of these hemodynamic changes in the ICA might be a potential noninvasive quantitative method of classifying treatment outcomes to follow up MMD patients after revascularization surgery.

11.4.3 The Vessel Remodeling Hemodynamic Analysis in the Circle of Willis

The intimal thickening is the specific pathological change of MMD, resulting in stenosis and/or occlusion of the ICA's terminal portion, MCA, and anterior cerebral artery. In an attempt to

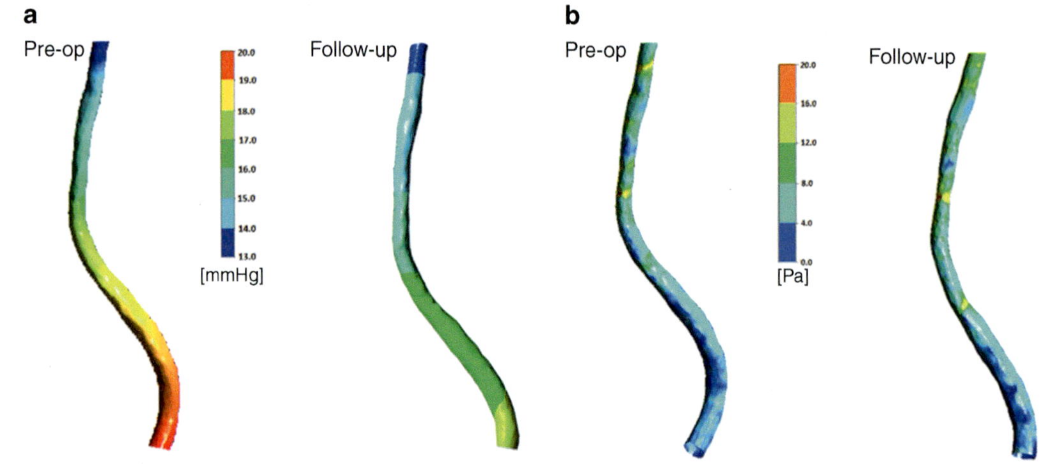

Fig. 11.7 Pressure and WSS distribution of illustrative cases in group A. (**a**) Pressure contours and (**b**) WSS contours of the surgically treated ICA in an illustrative case of group A preoperatively and at follow-up, representing the characteristic vessel remodeling of ICA. The ICA shrank, and the diameter and vascular tortuosity of the ICA trunk decreased. The WSS of the ICA trunk did not obviously change (Reproduced from Zhu F, Karunanithi K, Qian Y, Mao Y, Xu B, Gu Y, Zhu W, Chen L, Wang Y, Pan H, Liao Y, Morgan M. Assessing surgical treatment outcome following superficial temporal artery to middle cerebral artery bypass based on computational haemodynamic analysis. J Biomech. 2015; 48(15): 4053–58)

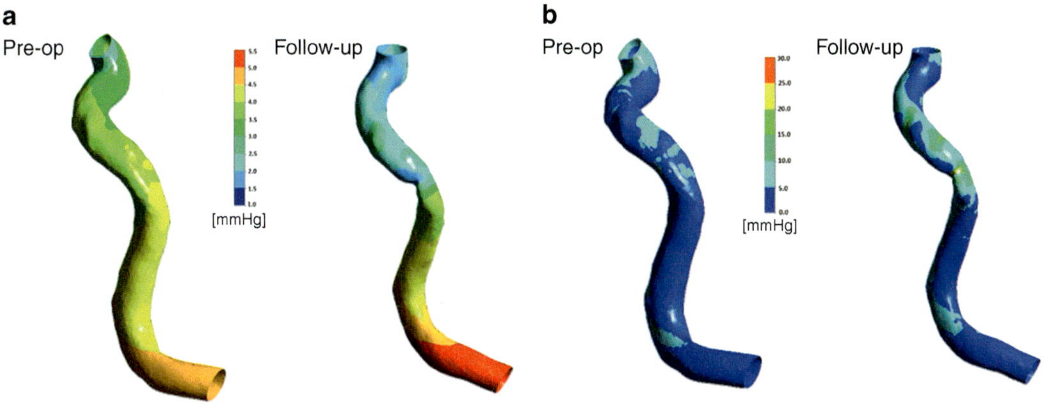

Fig. 11.8 Pressure and WSS distribution of an illustrative case of group C. (**a**) Pressure contours and (**b**) WSS contours of the treated ICA in one case of group C preoperatively and at follow-up. The pressure drops increased, and the diameter of the ICA did not obviously change; however, there was new and severe stenosis in the ICA trunk. The WSS in the stenotic portion of the ICA was higher than that in the preoperative model (Reproduced from Zhu F, Karunanithi K, Qian Y, Mao Y, Xu B, Gu Y, Zhu W, Chen L, Wang Y, Pan H, Liao Y, Morgan M. Assessing surgical treatment outcome following superficial temporal artery to middle cerebral artery bypass based on computational haemodynamic analysis. J Biomech. 2015; 48(15): 4053–58)

deliver blood to the ischemic brain, the collateral vessels form to compensate for the narrowing arteries and result in a hazy, film-like appearance that appears to be MMD on an angiogram. MMD is thus considered a dynamic cerebrovascular disease involving blood flow from the IC to the EC system. The involvement degree varies with the stage of MMD [18]. The "IC-EC conversion system" insufficiency may lead to cerebral ischemia, mostly. However, intracranial hemorrhage may also occur due to inadequate collateral vascular networks. EC-IC bypass is the preferred revascularization treatment for MMD complementing "IC-EC conversion." Both the cerebral infarction and/or the intracranial hemorrhage caused by MMD can be diminished by EC-IC bypass [18].

Hence, we assessed the ICA's hemodynamic and morphological modifications following bypass surgery through CFD technology quantitative microbiological risk assessment (QMRA). These techniques helped to explore the therapeutic mechanisms for revascularization surgery of MMD. Subgroup analysis, according to different configurations at the CoW, was performed. The pressure reduction in the bilateral ICAs was calculated at the inlet interface and the outlet's proximal end, between the preoperative and postoperative geometries' fixed coordinates, eliminating human error due to segmentation (Fig. 11.9).

CFD technology was applied to evaluate the pre- and postoperative pressure drop along the ICA. Besides, both the flow rate and the mean WSS through the ICA were quantified. The flow rate and pressure drop within the treated ICA were found to decline significantly following surgery (Fig. 11.10). The flow rate in the treated ICAs decreased by 14.83%, while the PDI decreased by 21.18%. This phenomenon agrees with the theory that bypass surgery is useful to complete the process of "IC-EC conversion" of MMD [18]. Once new collaterals following functional revascularization surgery are established, the ICA's hemodynamic function may be weakened, with lowered hemodynamic stress.

The CoW is an essential structure for creating collaterals or redundancies in cerebral circulation [19]. The hemodynamic changes within the ICA were analyzed according to the configurations of the CoW following bypass surgery. The contralateral ICA PDI decreased by 2.45% or 20.88% at follow-up in the groups with a complete or incomplete CoW, respectively. The more blood flow through the complete CoW may be the reason for less decrement of contralateral ICA PDI. Pressure drops in the treated ICA after

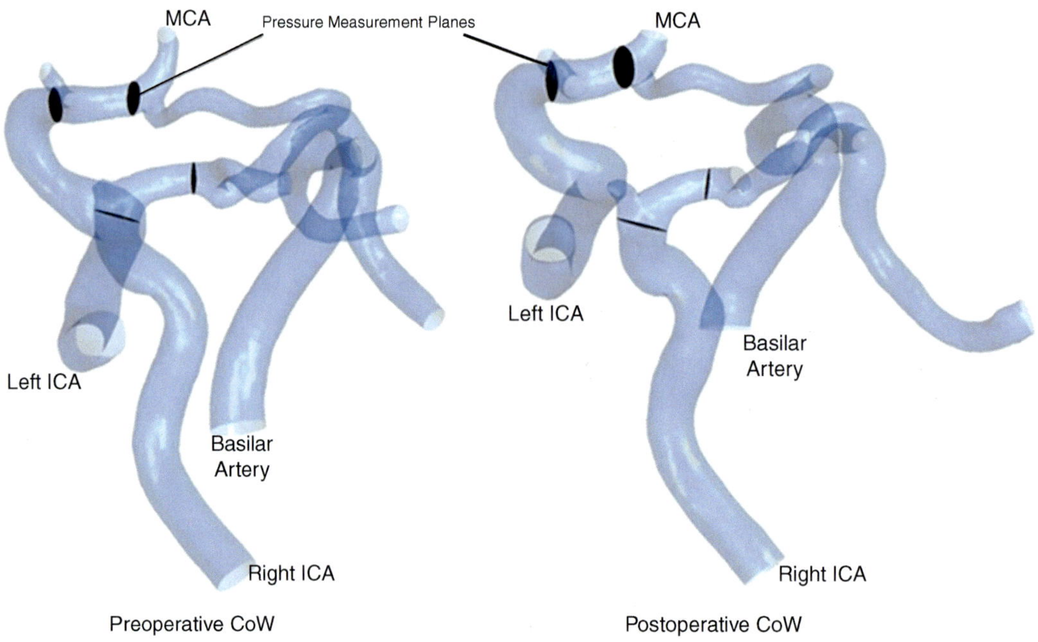

Fig. 11.9 Pressure measurement planes in the CoW

bypass may be matched to the contralateral ICA due to the CoW connection.

Vessel remodeling occurs in the treated ICA, with reductions in volumetric flow, vessel diameter, PDI, and mean WSS. This vessel remodeling pattern correlates with the dynamic "IC-EC conversion" nature of MMD. From a hemodynamic viewpoint, bypass surgery may help complete such an "IC-EC conversion" process. Successful bypass surgery can reduce the hemodynamic stress within the IC system. The PDI may be a potentially crucial biomechanical factor in the ICA's remodeling over time. The CoW configurations may influence the bypass surgery effect on the contralateral ICA.

11.5 Comments

Flow resistance might be regarded as a predictive parameter to predict bypass surgery outcomes regarding bypass patency. Vessel autoremodeling of the STA-MCA bypass graft was observed in the long-term follow-up. For the cases with a patent STA-MCA bypass at the long-term follow-up, the bypass's flow resistance is reduced, with a higher flow rate and increasingly uniform WSS. The initial bypass morphology significantly influences the vessel remodeling process. Both the curvature of the ipsilateral STA and the position of the STA-MCA bypass must be carefully assessed to optimize the revascularization surgery.

The ICA undergoes characteristic vessel remodeling after combined direct and indirect bypass surgery, decreasing the volume flow rate and PDI. Detailed analysis of hemodynamic changes in the ICA using CFD technology might be a potential noninvasive quantitative method to predict the bypass surgical outcomes of MMD at follow-up.

Our results supported the occurrence of "IC-EC conversion" following bypass surgery. After bypass surgery, the vessel remodeling within the ICA may reduce the pressure drop, volumetric flow the vessel diameter. The decrease in pressure drop and flow in the ipsilateral ICA is thought to be associated with a reduced hemodynamic burden, thus improving clinical outcomes.

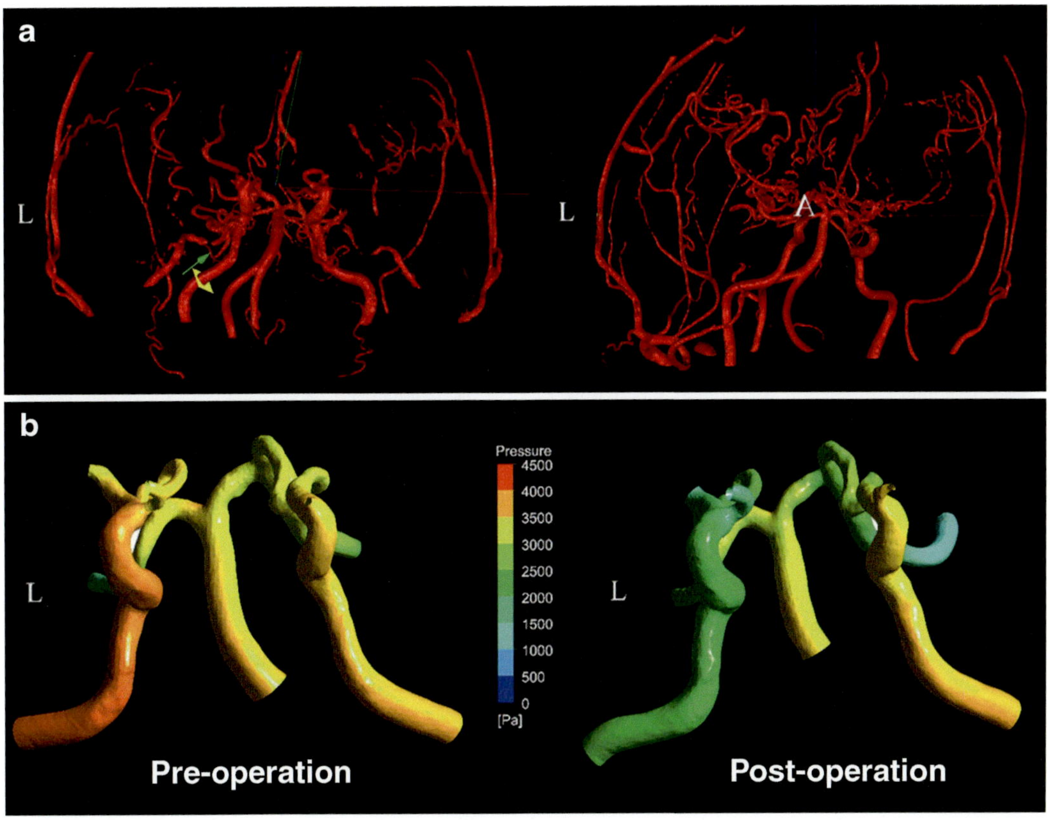

Fig. 11.10 Illustrative case. (**a**) Pre- and postoperative quantitative MRA post bypass surgery in the left hemisphere. The volumetric flow of the ICA decreased from 145 ml/min to 110 ml/min, with more than two-thirds of the MCA distribution area supplied by newly constructed vessel networks from the external carotid system. (**b**) Corresponding pressure contours showing that the pressure drop decreased in the bilateral ICAs (Reproduced from Zhu F, Qian Y, Xu B, Gu Y, Karunanithi K, Zhu W, Chen L, Mao Y, Morgan MK. Quantitative assessment of changes in hemodynamics of the internal carotid artery after bypass surgery for moyamoya disease. J Neurosurg. 2018; 129(3): 677–83)

Moreover, the CoW configurations will influence the bypass surgical effect on the contralateral ICA. Therefore, we advocate continuous long-term hemodynamic monitoring for the contralateral hemisphere in the progressive MMD.

References

1. Lee BK. Computational fluid dynamics in cardiovascular disease. Korean Circ J. 2011;41(8):423–30.
2. Farnoush A, Avolio A, Qian Y. A growth model of saccular aneurysms based on hemodynamic and morphologic discriminant parameters for risk of rupture. J Clin Neurosci. 2014;21(9):1514–9.
3. Lim CT, Goh JCH, editors. Biomedical engineering analysis of the rupture risk of cerebral aneurysms: flow comparison of three small pre-ruptured versus six large unruptured cases. Berlin: Springer; 2009. p. 1600–3.
4. Qian Y, Takao H, Umezu M, Murayama Y. Risk analysis of unruptured aneurysms using computational fluid dynamics technology: preliminary results. AJNR Am J Neuroradiol. 2011;32(10):1948–55.
5. Sen Y, Qian Y, Avolio A, Morgan M. Image segmentation methods for intracranial aneurysm haemodynamic research. J Biomech. 2014;47(5):1014–9.
6. Shojima M, Morita A, Kimura T, Oshima M, Kin T, Saito N. Computational fluid dynamic simulation of a giant basilar tip aneurysm with eventual rupture after Hunterian ligation. World Neurosurg. 2014;82(3–4):535.
7. Cheng SW, Lam ES, Fung GS, Ho P, Ting AC, Chow KW. A computational fluid dynamic study of stent

graft remodeling after endovascular repair of thoracic aortic dissections. J Vasc Surg. 2008;48(2):303–9. 309–10
8. Alaraj A, Amin-Hanjani S, Shakur SF, Aletich VA, Ivanov A, Carlson AP, Oh G, Charbel FT. Quantitative assessment of changes in cerebral arteriovenous malformation hemodynamics after embolization. Stroke. 2015;46(4):942–7.
9. Seol HJ, Shin DC, Kim YS, Shim EB, Kim SK, Cho BK, Wang KC. Computational analysis of hemodynamics using a two-dimensional model in moyamoya disease. J Neurosurg Pediatr. 2010;5(3):297–301.
10. Charbel FT, Misra M, Clarke ME, Ausman JI. Computer simulation of cerebral blood flow in moyamoya and the results of surgical therapies. Clin Neurol Neurosurg. 1997;99(Suppl 2):S68–73.
11. Kim T, Bang JS, Kwon OK, Hwang G, Kim JE, Kang HS, Cho WS, Moon JU, Oh CW. Morphology and related hemodynamics of the internal carotid arteries of moyamoya patients. Acta Neurochir. 2015;157(5):755–61.
12. Karunanithi K, Han C, Lee CJ, Shi W, Duan L, Qian Y. Identification of a hemodynamic parameter for assessing treatment outcome of EDAS in Moyamoya disease. J Biomech. 2015;48(2):304–9.
13. Zhu FP, Zhang Y, Higurashi M, Xu B, Gu YX, Mao Y, Morgan MK, Qian Y. Haemodynamic analysis of vessel remodelling in STA-MCA bypass for Moyamoya disease and its impact on bypass patency. J Biomech. 2014;47(8):1800–5.
14. Zhu F, Qian Y, Xu B, Gu Y, Karunanithi K, Zhu W, Chen L, Mao Y, Morgan MK. Quantitative assessment of changes in hemodynamics of the internal carotid artery after bypass surgery for moyamoya disease. J Neurosurg. 2018;129(3):677–83.
15. Zhu F, Karunanithi K, Qian Y, Mao Y, Xu B, Gu Y, Zhu W, Chen L, Wang Y, Pan H, Liao Y, Morgan M. Assessing surgical treatment outcome following superficial temporal artery to middle cerebral artery bypass based on computational haemodynamic analysis. J Biomech. 2015;48(15):4053–8.
16. Kim M, Taulbee DB, Tremmel M, Meng H. Comparison of two stents in modifying cerebral aneurysm hemodynamics. Ann Biomed Eng. 2008;36(5):726–41.
17. Matsushima Y, Inaba Y. Moyamoya disease in children and its surgical treatment. Introduction of a new surgical procedure and its follow-up angiograms. Childs Brain. 1984;11(3):155–70.
18. Fujimura M, Tominaga T. Current status of revascularization surgery for Moyamoya disease: special consideration for its 'internal carotid-external carotid (IC-EC) conversion' as the physiological reorganization system. Tohoku J Exp Med. 2015;236(1):45–53.
19. Alnaes MS, Isaksen J, Mardal KA, Romner B, Morgan MK, Ingebrigtsen T. Computation of hemodynamics in the circle of Willis. Stroke. 2007;38(9):2500–5.

12 Functional Magnetic Resonance Imaging Study of Cerebral Revascularization in Moyamoya Disease

Yu Lei and Yuxiang Gu

Abstract

First, functional magnetic resonance imaging (fMRI) is not associated with the surgical techniques during anastomosis, and patency of the graft is decided by daily practice rather than a preoperative fMRI scan. Thus, fMRI studies of cerebral revascularization are confronted with huge challenges in clinical practice. In our center, fMRI has been applied to surgical revascularization for almost ten years, and we have found some indications and possibilities to unlock its value. Since fMRI studies of cerebral revascularization have mainly focused on bypass surgery for Moyamoya disease, we briefly describe their recent advances based on our researches.

Keywords

Blood oxygenation level-dependent signal Extracranial-intracranial bypass · Functional magnetic resonance imaging · Low-frequency fluctuations · Moyamoya disease Revascularization

Y. Lei · Y. Gu (✉)
Huashan Hospital, Shanghai Medical College, Fudan University, Shanghai, China

12.1 Preface

First, functional magnetic resonance imaging (fMRI) is not associated with the surgical techniques during anastomosis, and patency of the graft is decided by daily practice rather than a preoperative fMRI scan. Thus, fMRI studies of cerebral revascularization are confronted with huge challenges in clinical practice. In our center, fMRI has been applied to surgical revascularization for almost 10 years, and we have found some indications and possibilities to unlock its value. In the following text, detailed and reasonable suggestions of its applications and notes based on our experiences are proposed for discussion.

12.2 Introduction

During the fMRI scan, the blood oxygenation level-dependent (BOLD) signals of the whole brain are collected. Both rest and task conditions are commonly assessed in fMRI studies. However, resting-state fMRI is more suitable than task fMRI for patients with verbal, motor, or mental dysfunctions; thus, resting-state fMRI is used more frequently in patients with cerebrovascular diseases (CVDs).

Among the BOLD signals, the amplitude of low-frequency fluctuations (ALFFs) (<0.1 Hz) was collected. Numerous studies have proven that ALFFs arise primarily from spontaneous

Y. Mao et al. (eds.), *Surgical Atlas of Cerebral Revascularization*,
https://doi.org/10.1007/978-981-16-0374-7_12

fluctuations of neuronal activity and brain physiology, and provide insight into the brain's intrinsic functional architecture [1]. Using graphical theoretical analysis of resting-state fMRI, researchers have proved that the whole brain is functionally connected and responds to high-level cognitive demand [2]. Thus, BOLD fMRI is considered a promising tool to detect abnormal brain functions.

Although neuropsychological tests are deemed necessary to evaluate cognitive function, their application in CVD is limited because of their ceiling and floor effects and the requirement of physical and mental cooperation. Numerous studies have found a close relation between BOLD fMRI parameters and neuropsychological test scores and recommend the use of BOLD fMRI to map the spatial distribution of brain regions with aberrant functions [3]. In summary, fMRI is deemed a promising tool to evaluate brain status before and after cerebral revascularization and a candidate indicator for surgical decision-making.

12.3 Details of the Procedure

Imaging acquisition parameters and preprocessing procedures are not identical across different MRI systems and should be adjusted accordingly. Nevertheless, they have common factors that should be considered, which are listed below.

Referring to data acquisition, higher field systems definitely result in higher-resolution images, but the clinical benefits are not definite, and patient safety is not guaranteed, especially for those with skull patches from surgical cranioplasty. Therefore, a 3.0-Tesla MRI system is recommended for scanning. Then, patients should keep their eyes closed and remain clearly conscious during the scan. Eye shields are recommended for those with poor compliance. In addition, the scanning sequences should be arranged carefully, and the BOLD data should not be acquired too late in case the patients fall asleep.

For data preprocessing, several semiautomatic toolboxes based on MATLAB that are free and easy to use are available on the market. We usually use the Data Processing Assistant for Resting-State fMRI (DPARSF), Statistical Parametric Mapping (SPM; http://www.fil.ion.ucl.ac.uk/spm), and the Resting-State fMRI Data Analysis Toolkit (REST; http://rest.restfmri.net) in our daily work [4, 5]. In detail, we discarded the first 10 volumes due to the initial MRI signal instability. The remaining volumes were then subjected to slice timing correction and realignment for head motion correction. Using least-squares minimization, we realigned the functional volumes, without higher-order corrections for spin history. The imaging data were then normalized to the Montreal Neurological Institute template, warped to 3-mm isotropic voxels, and smoothed with a 4-mm full-width half-maximum Gaussian kernel. The linear trend subtraction and temporal filtering (0.01–0.08 Hz) were performed on each voxel's time series to reduce the effect of low-frequency drifts and high-frequency noise [6]. Subsequent analyses refer to the aims of different studies.

12.4 Advances

Since fMRI studies of cerebral revascularization have mainly focused on bypass surgery for Moyamoya disease (MMD), we briefly describe their recent advances as examples.

The brain functions as a whole, and the associated abnormalities in CVD can be caused by dysfunction of either regional neurons or global neural interactions. fMRI studies are subdivided into three levels: microscale (network nodes), middle scale (subnetwork), and large scale (whole network). Brain dysfunction of adult MMD has been investigated at these three levels.

In microscale studies, the parameter of ALFFs was adopted [7]. First, abnormal intrinsic functional activity was detected in adult MMD patients. Then, the ALFF patterns were found to change within many brain regions with progressive cognitive decline. Notably, we found that the most remarkable differences in ALFF occurred in regions such as the anterior cingulate cortex (ACC), prefrontal cortex (PFC), and right supplemental motor area (SMA). We also found that the right middle frontal gyrus (MFG), right SMA, bilateral ACC, and orbitofrontal gyrus (OFG) showed the most significant correlation with Mini-Mental State Examination (MMSE) scores. Furthermore, a positive correlation with MMSE scores was found in the bilateral superior parietal lobe, inferior parietal lobe (IPL), and left caudate nucleus, while a negative correlation was found in the bilateral precuneus (PCu) (Fig. 12.1).

Postoperative brain function changes have also been investigated in adult MMD at the nodal level [8]. Compared with controls, adult MMD patients exhibited a significant decrease in regional ALFFs, mainly in the frontal and parietal lobes. However, ALFFs increased significantly in some prefrontal areas (Fig. 12.2a). Afterward, these abnormal regions' ALFF values were correlated with executive function (MES-EX scores) (Fig. 12.2b). Significant positive correlations were mainly observed in the parietal lobe, including the bilateral IPL, the PCu, and the posterior cingulate cortex (PCC), as well as the anterior PFC. Significant negative correlations were noticed in the frontal lobe, such as the bilateral dorsolateral prefrontal cortex (DLPFC) and some subcortical regions [8].

Next, the individual ALFF maps before surgery and at the 6-month follow-up were compared and analyzed. The results indicated that only the left PCu, bilateral PCC, and right DLPFC demonstrated remarkable postoperative ALFF changes (Fig. 12.3). The follow-up changes (△)

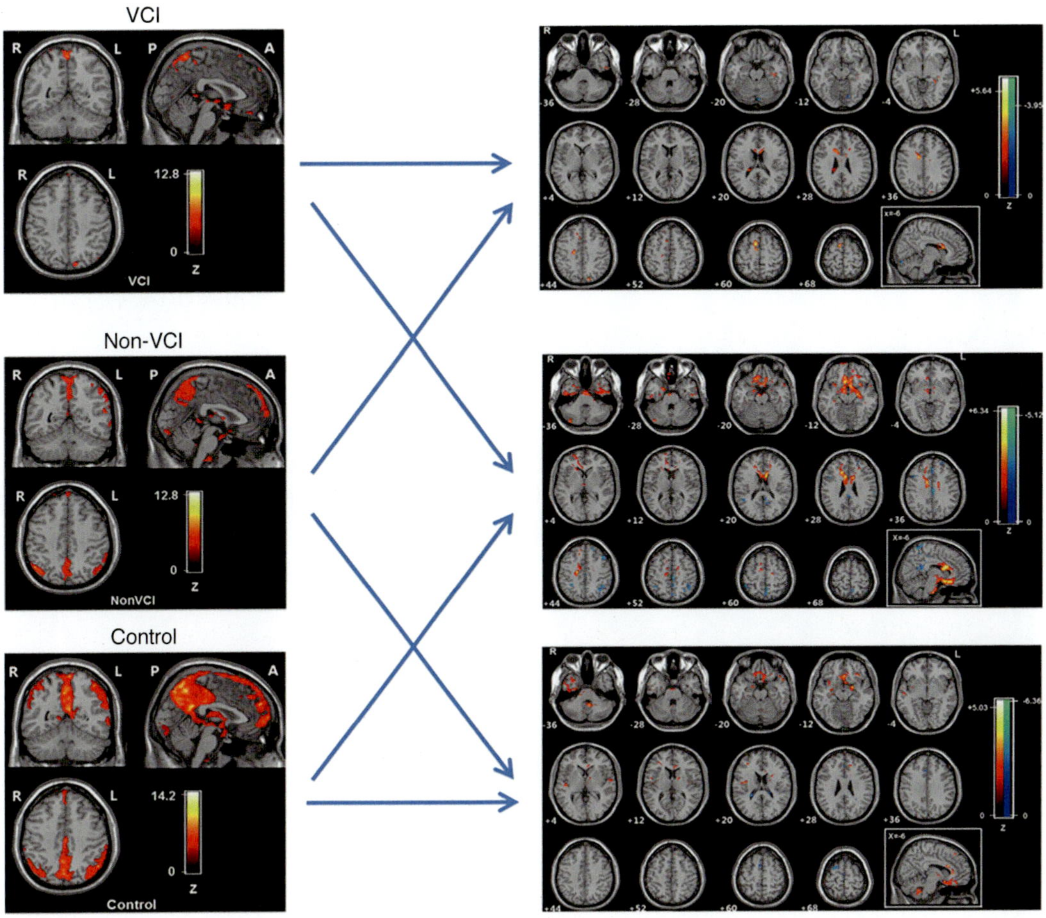

Fig. 12.1 The regional ALFF patterns and a comparison of functional deterioration among adult patients with MMD and vascular cognitive impairment (VCI), adult patients with MMD and intact cognition (non-VCI), and controls (Modified from Lei Y, Li Y, Ni W, Jiang H, Yang Z, Guo Q, Gu Y, Mao Y. Spontaneous brain activity in adult patients with moyamoya disease: a resting-state fMRI study. Brain Res. 2014; 1546: 27–33)

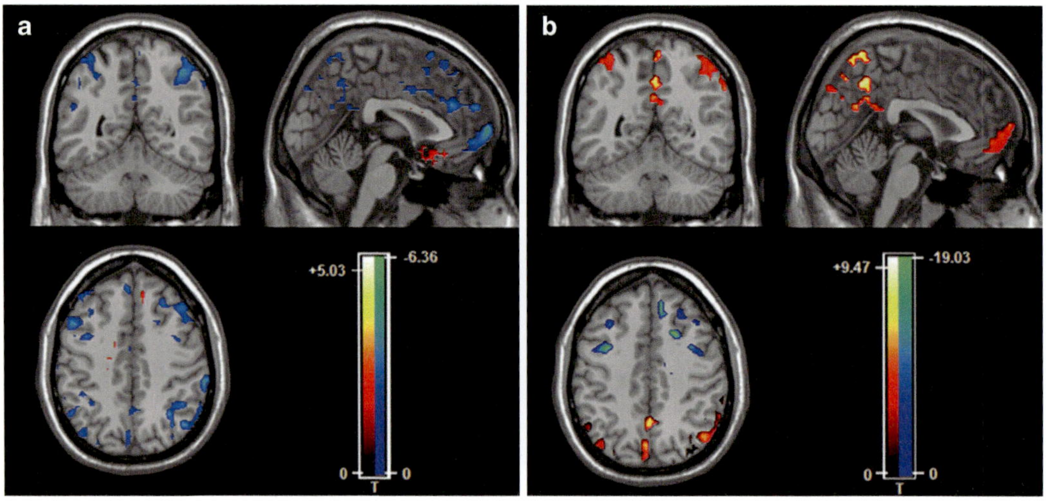

Fig. 12.2 The regional ALFF patterns of MMD patients compared to those of controls (**a**); Correlation maps of executive function and regional ALFF values within the abnormal regions (**b**) (Reproduced from Lei Y, Li YJ, Guo QH, Liu XD, Liu Z, Ni W, Su JB, Yang H, Jiang HQ, Xu B, Gu YX, Mao Y. Postoperative executive function in adult moyamoya disease: a preliminary study of its functional anatomy and behavioral correlates. J Neurosurg. 2017; 126(2): 527–536)

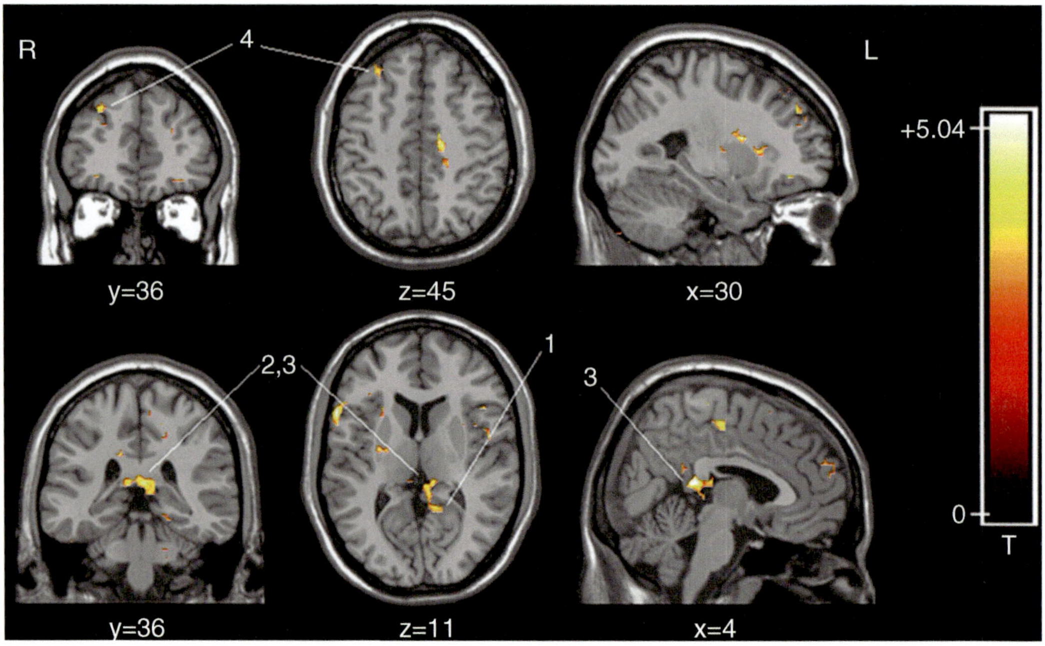

Fig. 12.3 The paired-sample t-test shows the regions with significant ALFF changes after cerebral revascularization. The left PCu (1), bilateral posterior cingulate cortex (2), and right DLPFC (3) were generated (Reproduced from Lei Y, Li YJ, Guo QH, Liu XD, Liu Z, Ni W, Su JB, Yang H, Jiang HQ, Xu B, Gu YX, Mao Y. Postoperative executive function in adult moyamoya disease: a preliminary study of its functional anatomy and behavioral correlates. J Neurosurg. 2017; 126(2): 527–536)

in hemodynamics, ALFFs, and MES-EX scores were calculated and compared based on brain lobes. The results showed significant positive correlations only presented in the right frontal lobe between postoperative radiological changes and cognitive improvement (Fig. 12.4). Finally, the right DLPFC was found to be the only node that met all the above standards. Therefore, we concluded that the nodal changes of the right DLPFC might be the primary marker for predicting postoperative cognitive improvement, while the nodal changes of the left PCu and bilateral PCC may act as autoregulation to topological changes [8].

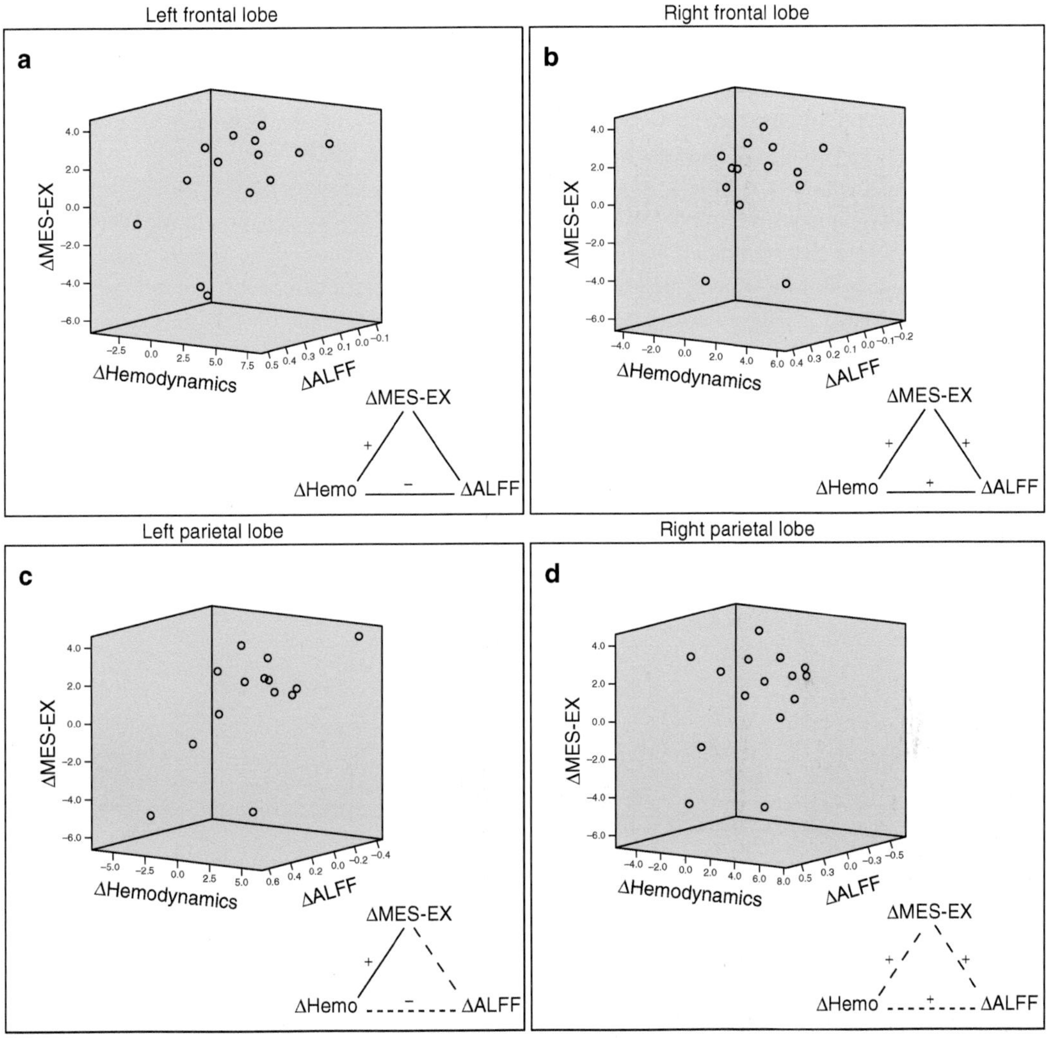

Fig. 12.4 Three-dimensional scatter diagrams showing the correlation between each pair of follow-up changes (ALFFs, hemodynamics, and MES-EX scores) in the left frontal (**a**), right frontal (**b**), left parietal (**c**), and right parietal (**d**) lobes. The solid lines indicate significant correlations, and the dashed lines indicate statistically insignificant correlations (Reproduced from Lei Y, Li YJ, Guo QH, Liu XD, Liu Z, Ni W, Su JB, Yang H, Jiang HQ, Xu B, Gu YX, Mao Y. Postoperative executive function in adult moyamoya disease: a preliminary study of its functional anatomy and behavioral correlates. J Neurosurg. 2017; 126(2): 527–536)

Referring to middle-scale studies, the functional networks were investigated [6]. Regional neural interactions are organized in response to cognitive demands. For example, the executive control network (ECN) mainly includes the DLPFC, posterior parietal gyrus, and MFG/superior frontal gyrus (SFG); the default mode network (DMN) mainly involves the PCC/PCu, medial PFC, angular gyrus (AG), and medial temporal gyrus; and the salience network (SN) mainly includes the ventrolateral PFC, ACC, and anterior insula. In our previous study, the parameter of regional homogeneity (ReHo) was adopted for network analysis. The physical significance of this parameter is to test the regional synchrony of spontaneous BOLD fMRI signals. Primarily, we found that compared with normal controls, patients with MMD presented with significantly decreased ReHo values in the left DLPFC, right medial SFG, right medial OFG, left IPL, right SFG, and right SMA and significantly increased ReHo values in the left middle temporal gyrus (MTG) (Fig. 12.5).

Afterward, the mean ReHo values of the ECN, DMN, and SN were calculated and compared between patients with MMD and normal controls (Fig. 12.6). The results showed that patients with MMD exhibited significantly decreased ReHo values in the right PCu, left medial SFG, right medial OFG of the DMN, the IPL, SFG, and DLPFC of the right ECN, the IPL, and DLPFC of the left ECN, and the right SMA and left MFG of the SN compared to controls. Furthermore, these networks all exhibited a pattern of decreasing mean ReHo values with disease severity. However, only the ECN presented a significant decrease (Fig. 12.7).

Next, the network ReHo values were correlated with executive function in MMD (MES-EX and TMT-B scores). The results indicated that only the ReHo values of the bilateral ECNs exhibited significant correlations with TMT-B and MES-EX scores (Figs. 12.8 and 12.9).

Referring to large-scale studies, the graphical theory of fMRI indicates that the entire brain network is organized as a whole and responds to

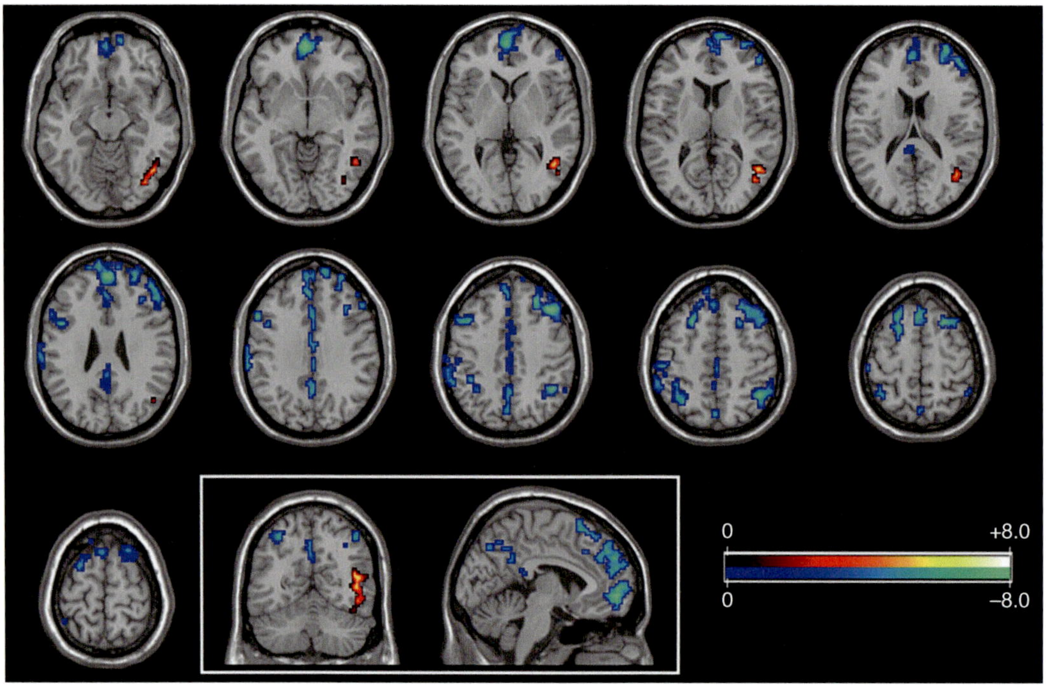

Fig. 12.5 Whole-brain ReHo differences between patients with MMD and normal controls. The statistical significance threshold was set at a corrected $p < 0.05$ (Reproduced from Lei Y, Su J, Jiang H, Guo Q, Ni W, Yang H, Gu Y, Mao Y. Aberrant regional homogeneity of resting-state executive control, default mode, and salience networks in adult patients with moyamoya disease. Brain Imaging Behav. 2017; 11(1): 176–184)

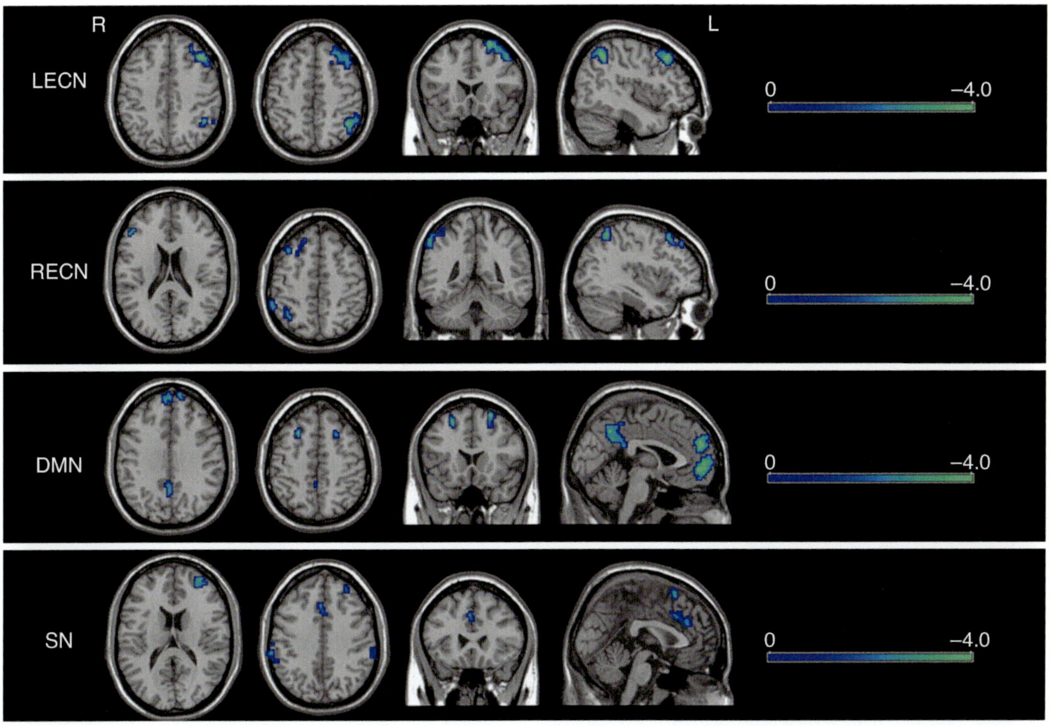

Fig. 12.6 Network ReHo differences between patients with MMD and normal controls. The statistical significance threshold was set at a corrected $p < 0.05$ (Reproduced from Lei Y, Su J, Jiang H, Guo Q, Ni W, Yang H, Gu Y, Mao Y. Aberrant regional homogeneity of resting-state executive control, default mode, and salience networks in adult patients with moyamoya disease. Brain Imaging Behav. 2017; 11(1):176–184)

cognitive demands efficiently. This "small-world" organization requires different brain regions to behave in certain patterns at a minimal cost for most effective information processing. Measurements of large-scale networks include network segregation, integration, and small-worldness.

The results indicated that patients with cognitive impairment (VCI group), patients with intact cognition (nonVCI group), and healthy controls exhibited significant differences in network segregation (local efficiency, clustering coefficient, and modularity) at all threshold levels (Fig. 12.10). Compared to both the nonVCI and the control groups, the VCI group exhibited a trend toward decreased local efficiency and clustering coefficients and increased modularity. Furthermore, in a wide sparsity range, the three groups exhibited significant differences in local efficiency and clustering coefficients, with a trend of controls > nonVCI > VCI.

Referring to the network integration of global path length and efficiency, the three groups presented significant differences at all threshold levels. Similar to network segregation, the VCI group exhibited a trend toward decreased global efficiency and increased path length compared with the nonVCI and control groups. In addition, only a small range of global efficiency was significantly different among the three groups in the defined sparsity range.

Referring to network small-worldness, significant differences among the three groups were found at all threshold levels. Specifically, the three groups exhibited a consistent decreasing trend from the controls to the nonVCI group and then to the VCI group. In addition, the three groups exhibited statistically insignificant differences in the whole sparsity range.

Next, the interregional differences in small-world properties among the three groups were calculated and compared (Fig. 12.11). At a

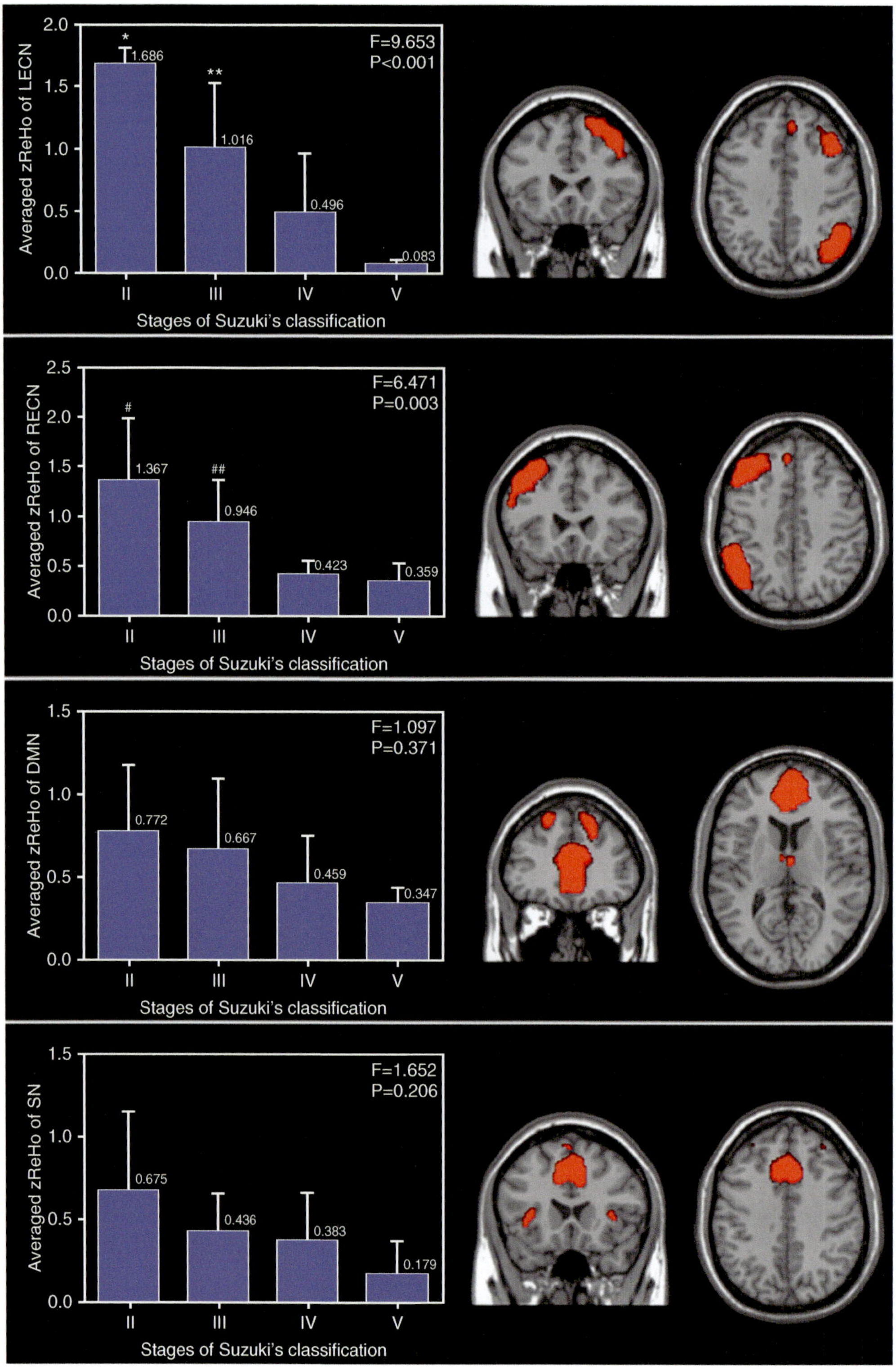

Fig. 12.7 Comparison of network ReHo differences among different disease Suzuki stages (Reproduced from Lei Y, Su J, Jiang H, Guo Q, Ni W, Yang H, Gu Y, Mao Y. Aberrant regional homogeneity of resting-state executive control, default mode, and salience networks in adult patients with moyamoya disease. Brain Imaging Behav. 2017; 11(1):176–184)

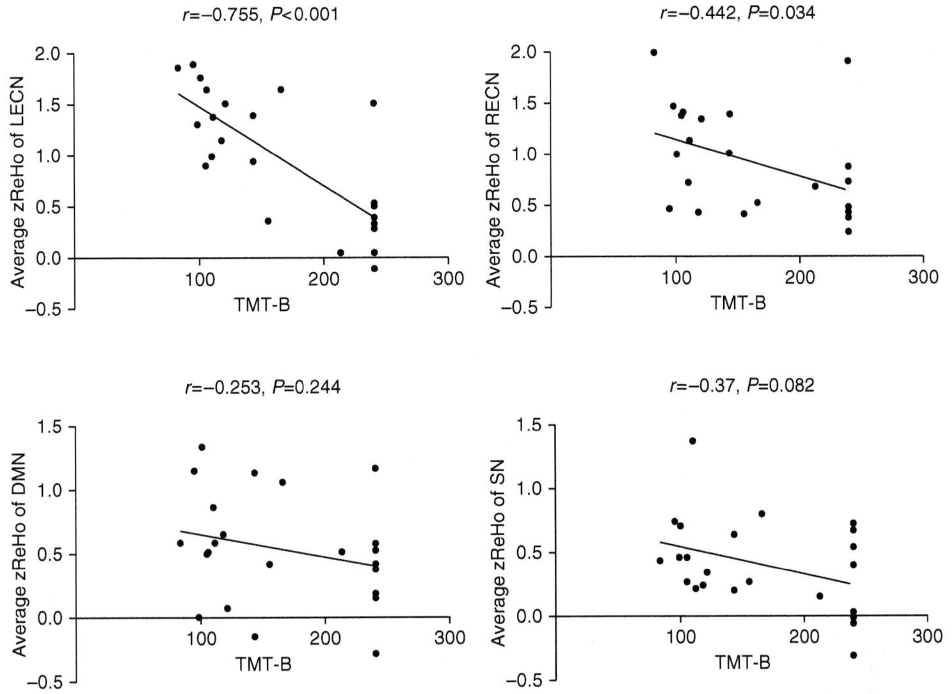

Fig. 12.8 Correlations between network ReHo values and TMT-B scores of executive functions (Reproduced from Lei Y, Su J, Jiang H, Guo Q, Ni W, Yang H, Gu Y, Mao Y. Aberrant regional homogeneity of resting-state executive control, default mode, and salience networks in adult patients with moyamoya disease. Brain Imaging Behav. 2017; 11(1): 176–184)

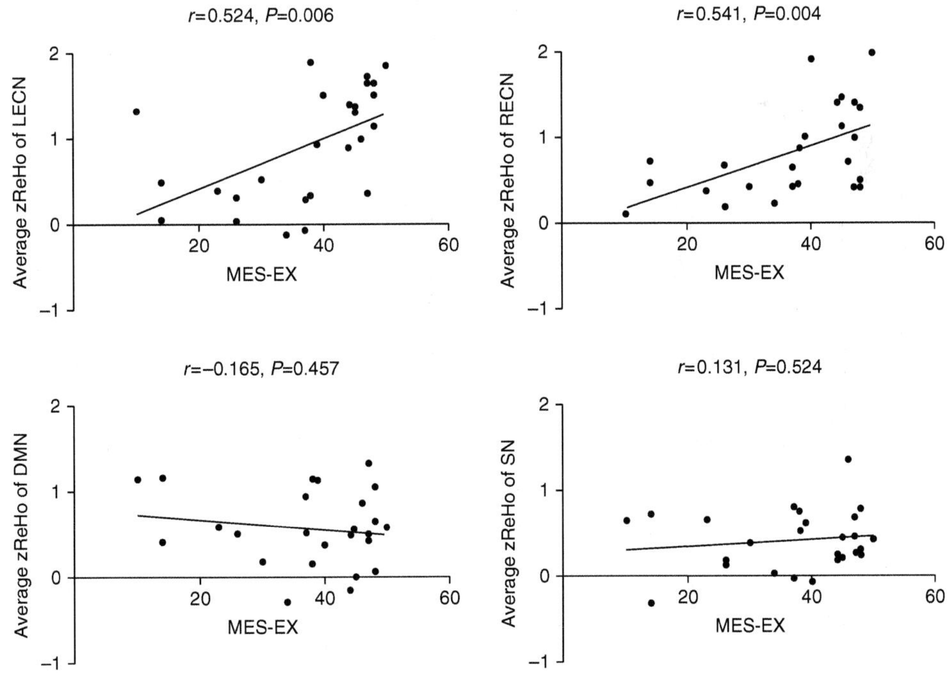

Fig. 12.9 Correlations between network ReHo values and MES-EX scores of executive functions (Reproduced from Lei Y, Su J, Jiang H, Guo Q, Ni W, Yang H, Gu Y, Mao Y. Aberrant regional homogeneity of resting-state executive control, default mode, and salience networks in adult patients with moyamoya disease. Brain Imaging Behav. 2017; 11(1): 176–184)

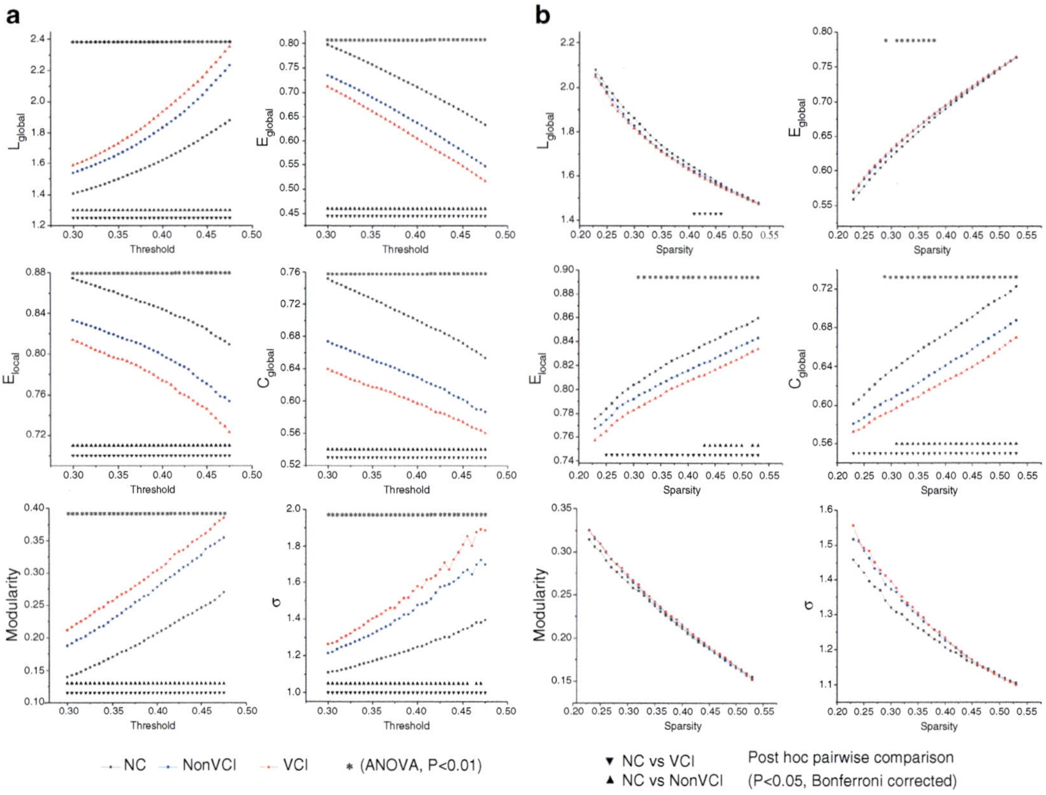

Fig. 12.10 Differences in network topologic metrics among the three groups of patients with cognitive impairment (VCI), patients with intact cognition (nonVCI), and controls in the defined threshold (**a**) and sparsity (**b**) ranges (Reproduced from Lei Y, Song B, Chen L, Su J, Zhang X, Ni W, Yu Y, Xu B, Yu L, Gu Y, Mao Y. Reconfigured functional network dynamics in adult moyamoya disease: a resting-state fMRI study. Brain Imaging Behav. 2020; 14(3): 715–727)

selected threshold of 0.35 and sparsity of 0.4, widespread regional differences were noted in global efficiency, global path length, local efficiency, and clustering coefficients.

In recent years, the development of computing power has brought about new ideas and revolutionary changes in fMRI data processing and clinical application. Previously, the construction of an fMRI network was based on the hypothesis that the signal is stationary. However, real neuronal oscillations change frequently and respond in a timely manner to outside stimuli. Thus, the temporal dimension of neural activities should be analyzed rather than simply the average of the correlations of BOLD signals among different regions. Flexible fMRI networks involving the temporal dimension are termed dynamic brain networks. Our team has explored the dynamic brain network of adult patients with MMD in a preliminary fMRI study.

The dynamic functional connectivity was measured with the flexible parameter of connectivity number entropy (CNE). Similar to the previous measurement of the static network, the dynamic fMRI network was evaluated in three levels: in the micro, middle, and large scale.

The whole-brain and regional CNE differences were primarily calculated and compared among the three VCI, nonVCI, and control groups. The results showed that the controls exhibited significantly higher CNE values than the other two groups, with a pattern of VCI < nonVCI < controls (Fig. 12.12).

Next, regional CNE differences were compared between two of the three groups. The results showed that the VCI group exhibited sig-

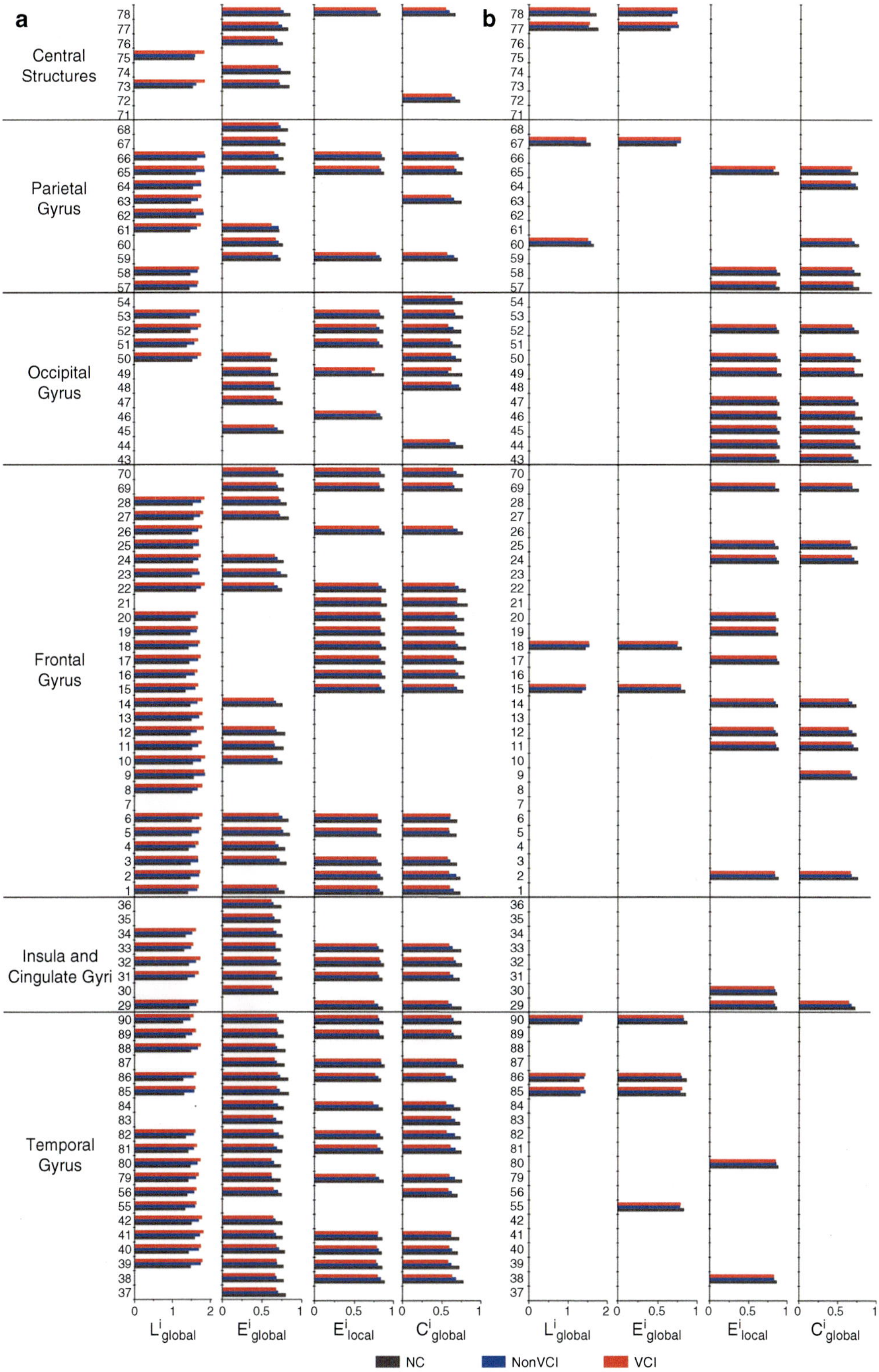

Fig. 12.11 Regional comparison of small-world metrics among the three groups of patients with cognitive impairment (VCI), patients with intact cognition (NonVCI), and normal controls (NC) (Reproduced from Lei Y, Song B, Chen L, Su J, Zhang X, Ni W, Yu Y, Xu B, Yu L, Gu Y, Mao Y. Reconfigured functional network dynamics in adult moyamoya disease: a resting-state fMRI study. Brain Imaging Behav. 2020; 14(3): 715–727)

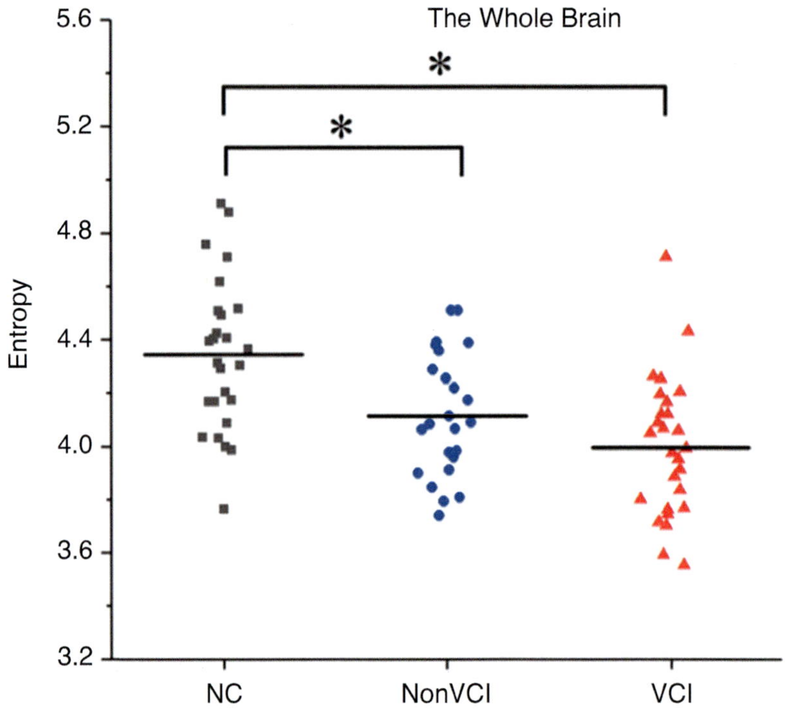

Fig. 12.12 Comparison of the whole-brain connectivity number entropy among the three groups of adult MMD patients with vascular cognitive impairment (VCI), adult MMD patients with intact cognition (nonVCI), and normal controls (NC) (Modified from Lei Y, Song B, Chen L, Su J, Zhang X, Ni W, Yu Y, Xu B, Yu L, Gu Y, Mao Y. Reconfigured functional network dynamics in adult moyamoya disease: a resting-state fMRI study. Brain Imaging Behav. 2020; 14(3): 715–727)

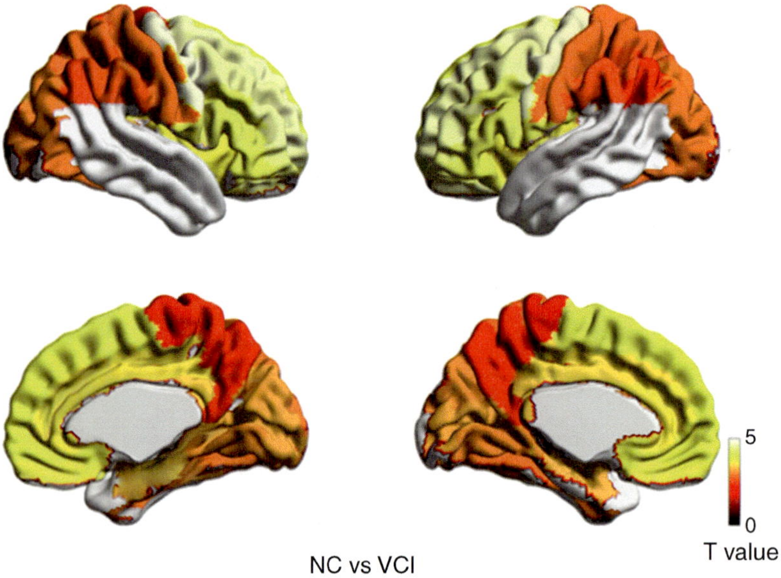

Fig. 12.13 Comparison of the regional CNE values between the normal controls (NC) and patients with vascular cognitive impairment (VCI) (Modified from Lei Y, Song B, Chen L, Su J, Zhang X, Ni W, Yu Y, Xu B, Yu L, Gu Y, Mao Y. Reconfigured functional network dynamics in adult moyamoya disease: a resting-state fMRI study. Brain Imaging Behav. 2020; 14(3): 715–727)

nificantly lower CNE values than the controls mainly in the bilateral OFG, DLPFC, MTG, inferior temporal gyrus, fusiform gyrus (FG), parahippocampal gyrus, AG, SMA, ACC, and regions involving the visual, auditory, and sensory areas (Fig. 12.13).

Moreover, patients with intact cognition exhibited significantly lower CNE values than the controls in parts of the OFG, right DLPFC, bilateral FG, lateral temporal cortices, left SMA, and parts of regions involving the visual, auditory, and sensory areas (Fig. 12.14). Interestingly,

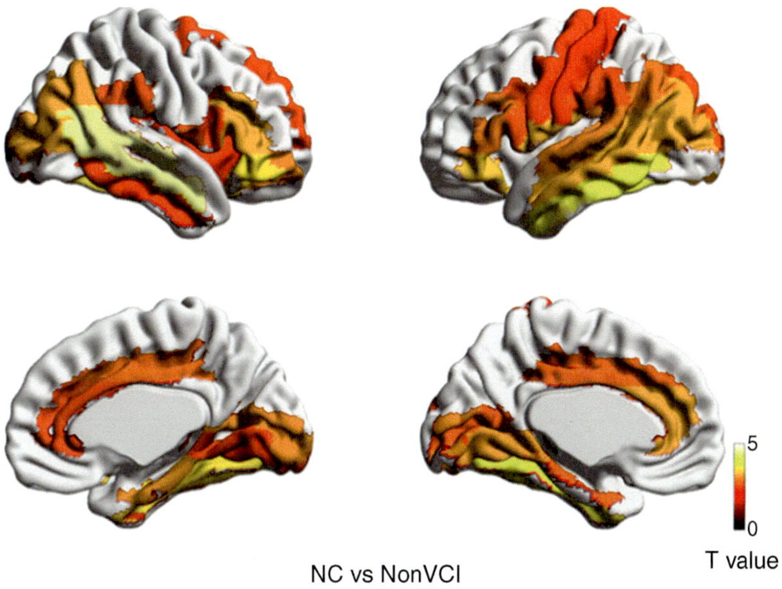

Fig. 12.14 Comparison of the regional CNE values between the controls and patients with intact cognition (Modified from Lei Y, Song B, Chen L, Su J, Zhang X, Ni W, Yu Y, Xu B, Yu L, Gu Y, Mao Y. Reconfigured functional network dynamics in adult moyamoya disease: a resting-state fMRI study. Brain Imaging Behav. 2020; 14(3):715–727)

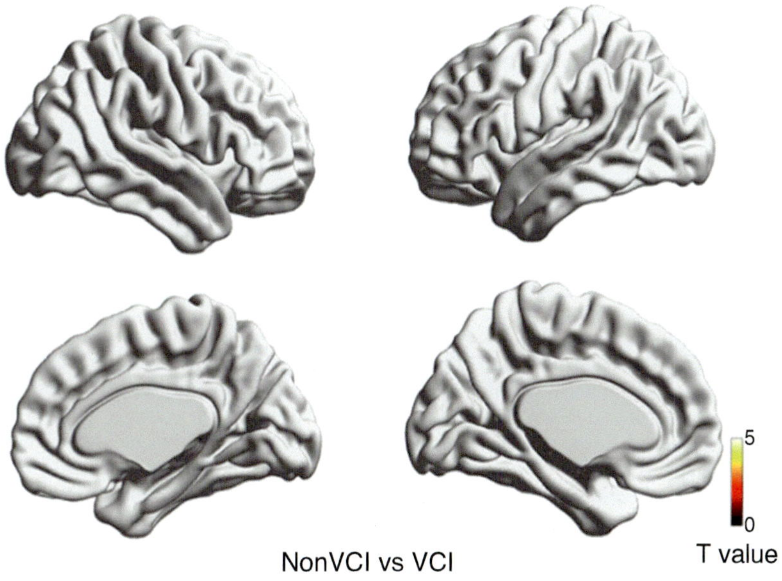

Fig. 12.15 Comparison of the regional CNE values between the patients with and without cognitive impairment (Modified from Lei Y, Song B, Chen L, Su J, Zhang X, Ni W, Yu Y, Xu B, Yu L, Gu Y, Mao Y. Reconfigured functional network dynamics in adult moyamoya disease: a resting-state fMRI study. Brain Imaging Behav. 2020; 14(3): 715–727)

no significant difference was noted between patients with and without cognitive impairment (Fig. 12.15).

Next, network CNE values were calculated and compared among the three groups. The results showed that both the DMN and ECN exhibited significantly different values among the three groups, while the differences in the SN were statistically insignificant. Nevertheless, all these networks exhibited a pattern of normal controls > nonVCI > VCI (Fig. 12.16).

Finally, the three groups' whole-brain CNE values were computed to investigate their dynamic changing patterns (Fig. 12.17). Normally, brain regions with high CNE values are termed functionally flexible regions, while regions with low CNE values are termed functionally specialized regions. The results showed

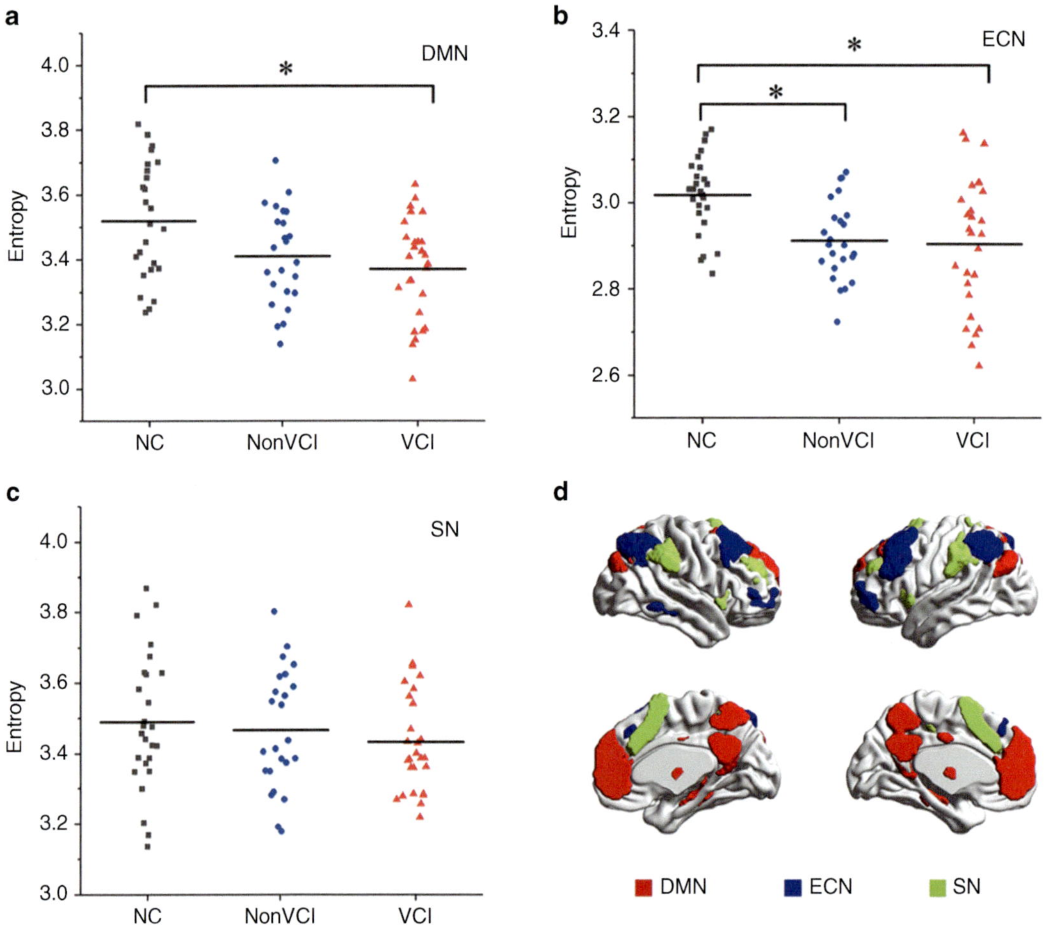

Fig. 12.16 Network CNE values were calculated and compared among patients with cognitive impairment (VCI), patients with intact cognition (NonVCI), and controls. A pattern of VCI < NonVCI < Normal controls (NC) was observed in all three networks of the default mode, (**a**), executive control (**b**) and salience networks (**c**). The horizontal line represents the mean value of each group. Black star stands for statistical significance ($p < 0.05$, Bonferroni corrected). (**d**) Atlases of functional regions of default mode (red), executive control (blue) and salience networks (green) (Reproduced from Lei Y, Song B, Chen L, Su J, Zhang X, Ni W, Yu Y, Xu B, Yu L, Gu Y, Mao Y. Reconfigured functional network dynamics in adult moyamoya disease: a resting-state fMRI study. Brain Imaging Behav. 2020; 14(3): 715–727)

that in healthy controls, flexible regions (termed as the 10 regions with the highest CNE values) were located in the FG, lateral temporal cortex, midcingulate gyrus, and parts of regions involving visual areas. Besides, specialized regions (termed as the 10 regions with the lowest CNE values) were noted in the left amygdala and pallidum, bilateral caudate and thalamus, and parts of regions involving semantic and sensory areas. However, the sequential order of these regions changes with disease progression (Fig. 12.18).

12.5 Comments

As one of the most important research hotspots in recent years, fMRI has been found to be sensitive and stable in detecting functional brain damage and recovery. We noted that in all three scales, at the nodal, network, and whole-brain levels, there are objective and quantitative fMRI parameters that can detect brain damage in CVDs such as MMD. Moreover, these fMRI parameters can be detected repeatedly and frequently after surgical

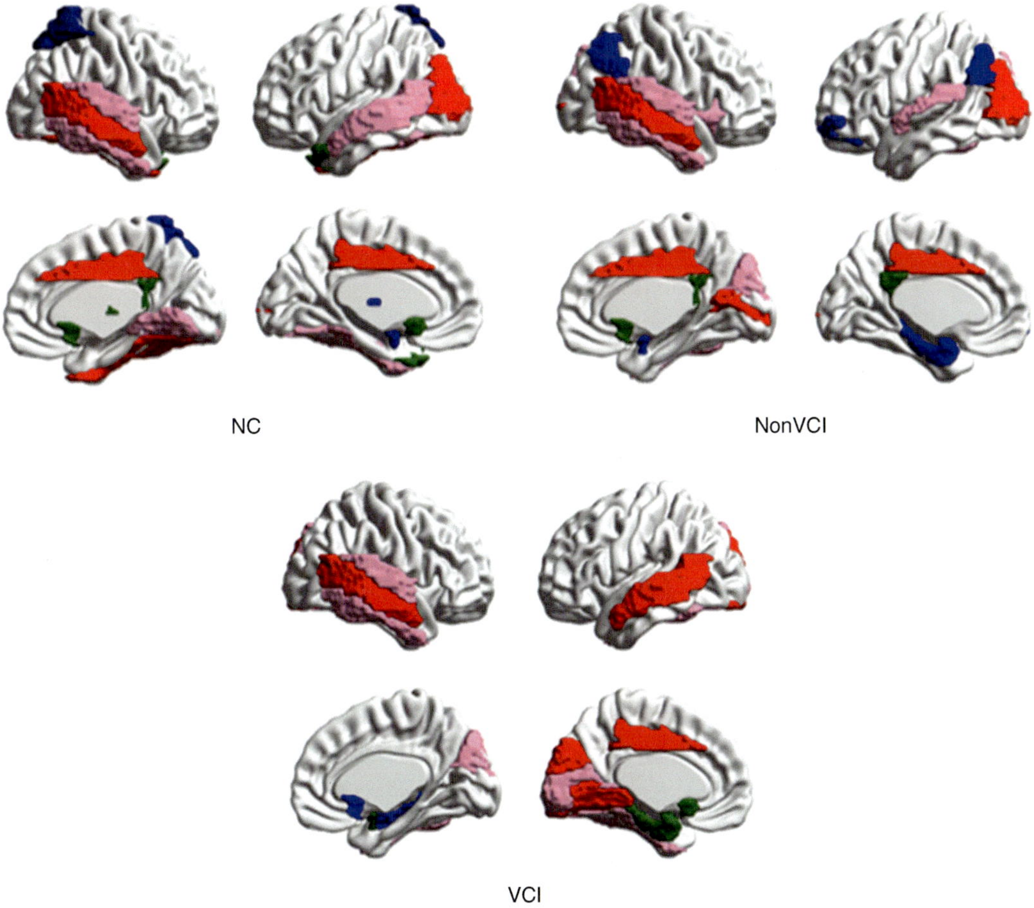

Fig. 12.17 Functionally flexible and specialized regions in the healthy controls (NC), MMD patients with intact cognition (NonVCI), and MMD patients with cognitive impairment (VCI) (Modified from Lei Y, Song B, Chen L, Su J, Zhang X, Ni W, Yu Y, Xu B, Yu L, Gu Y, Mao Y. Reconfigured functional network dynamics in adult moyamoya disease: a resting-state fMRI study. Brain Imaging Behav. 2020; 14(3): 715–727)

revascularization. Although fMRI is frequently limited by its difficulty in individualization, recent advances in both bulk data handling techniques and artificial intelligence technology may help provide promising solutions. In addition, fMRI techniques should be combined with structural MRI and other imaging modes to optimize the generation of an optimum evaluation system.

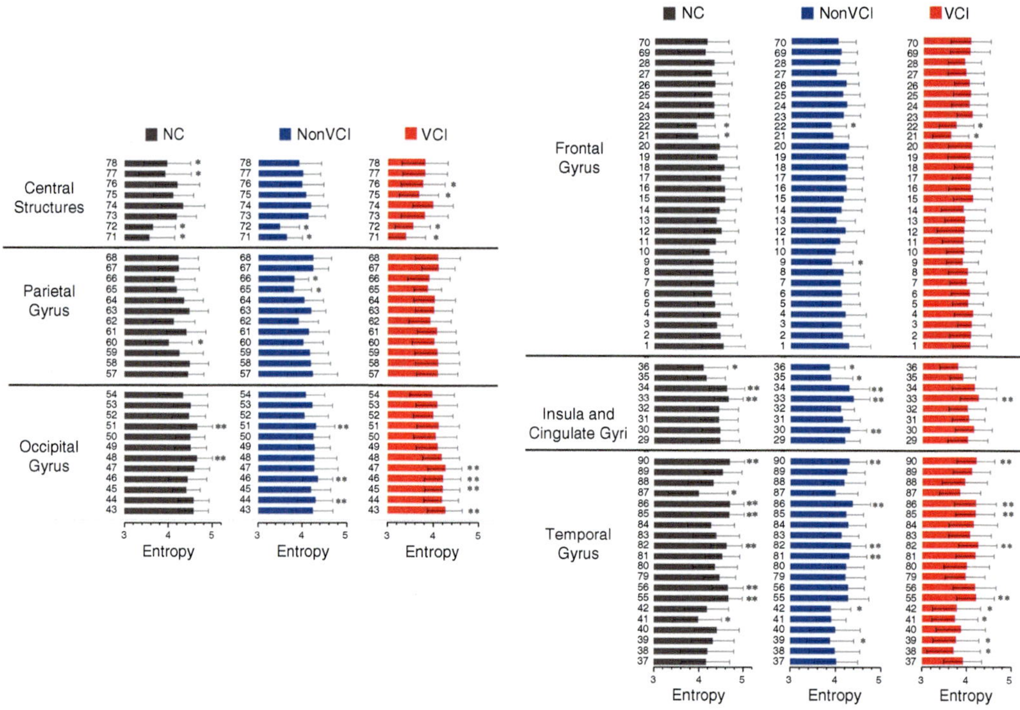

Fig. 12.18 Functionally flexible and specialized regions in patients with cognitive impairment (VCI), patients with intact cognition (NonVCI), and controls. (Modified from Lei Y, Song B, Chen L, Su J, Zhang X, Ni W, Yu Y, Xu B, Yu L, Gu Y, Mao Y. Reconfigured functional network dynamics in adult moyamoya disease: a resting-state fMRI study. Brain Imaging Behav. 2020; 14(3): 715–727)

References

1. Fox MD, Raichle ME. Spontaneous fluctuations in brain activity observed with functional magnetic resonance imaging. Nat Rev Neurosci. 2007;8(9):700–11.
2. Rubinov M, Sporns O. Complex network measures of brain connectivity: uses and interpretations. NeuroImage. 2010;52(3):1059–69.
3. Falkenberg LE, Westerhausen R, Specht K, Hugdahl K. Resting-state glutamate level in the anterior cingulate predicts blood-oxygen level-dependent response to cognitive control. Proc Natl Acad Sci U S A. 2012;109(13):5069–73.
4. Chao-Gan Y, Yu-Feng ZDPARSF. A MATLAB toolbox for "pipeline" data analysis of resting-state fMRI. Front Syst Neurosci. 2010;4:13.
5. Biswal B, Yetkin FZ, Haughton VM, Hyde JS. Functional connectivity in the motor cortex of resting human brain using echo-planar MRI. Magn Reson Med. 1995;34(4):537–41.
6. Lei Y, Su J, Jiang H, Guo Q, Ni W, Yang H, Gu Y, Mao Y. Aberrant regional homogeneity of resting-state executive control, default mode, and salience networks in adult patients with moyamoya disease. Brain Imaging Behav. 2017;11(1):176–84.
7. Lei Y, Li Y, Ni W, Jiang H, Yang Z, Guo Q, Gu Y, Mao Y. Spontaneous brain activity in adult patients with moyamoya disease: a resting-state fMRI study. Brain Res. 2014;1546:27–33.
8. Lei Y, Li YJ, Guo QH, Liu XD, Liu Z, Ni W, Su JB, Yang H, Jiang HQ, Xu B, Gu YX, Mao Y. Postoperative executive function in adult moyamoya disease: a preliminary study of its functional anatomy and behavioral correlates. J Neurosurg. 2017;126(2):527–36.

Perspective: The Topographic Model of Cerebral Revascularization

13

Xiang Zou, Jianping Song, Liang Chen, and Ying Mao

Abstract

Topology is a critical branch of mathematics. In topology, we focus on the invariance of change and ignore some details. The selection of the optimal surgical strategy is influenced by many variables, such as aneurysm morphology, size, vascular architecture, and even the surgeon's preference. However, from the perspective of topology, with the "topological neck" enclosing the inflow and/or outflow tract(s) on one side of the aneurysm, different aneurysms may be topologically equivalent in nature, regardless of the abovementioned variables.

Keywords

Intracranial aneurysm · Revascularization · Surgery · Topology

13.1 Introduction

Topology is a critical branch of mathematics. The idea underlying topology can be traced back to Gottfried Leibniz and was introduced by Johann Benedict Listing in the nineteenth century. Although topology is an abstract concept about a set theory, we can build vivid topological images. In topology, we focus on the invariance of change and ignore some details. For example, when we blow a balloon, no matter how much it is enlarged, the balloon is considered topologically equivalent unless an explosion occurs. Alternatively, a twisted piece of paper is topologically equivalent to a flat sheet of paper as long as it is not rolled and glued into a cylinder. Alternatively, a mug is topologically equivalent to a doughnut unless a bite has been taken out of the doughnut (Fig. 13.1). Topology can help us recognize the essential character of things.

Beings have multiplicity in structures. As we can ignore some details, such as size and shape, these structures can be divided into basic features from a topological view. The human brain has great intrinsic topological complexity, thus leading to its functional complexity. The vascular system also has a complex appearance, but its topological structure is elegantly simple. For instance, the circle of Willis is topologically equivalent to an inflatable floating ring but with holes (Fig. 13.1).

X. Zou · J. Song · L. Chen · Y. Mao (✉)
Huashan Hospital, Shanghai Medical College, Fudan University, Shanghai, China
e-mail: maoying@fudan.edu.cn

Y. Mao et al. (eds.), *Surgical Atlas of Cerebral Revascularization*,
https://doi.org/10.1007/978-981-16-0374-7_13

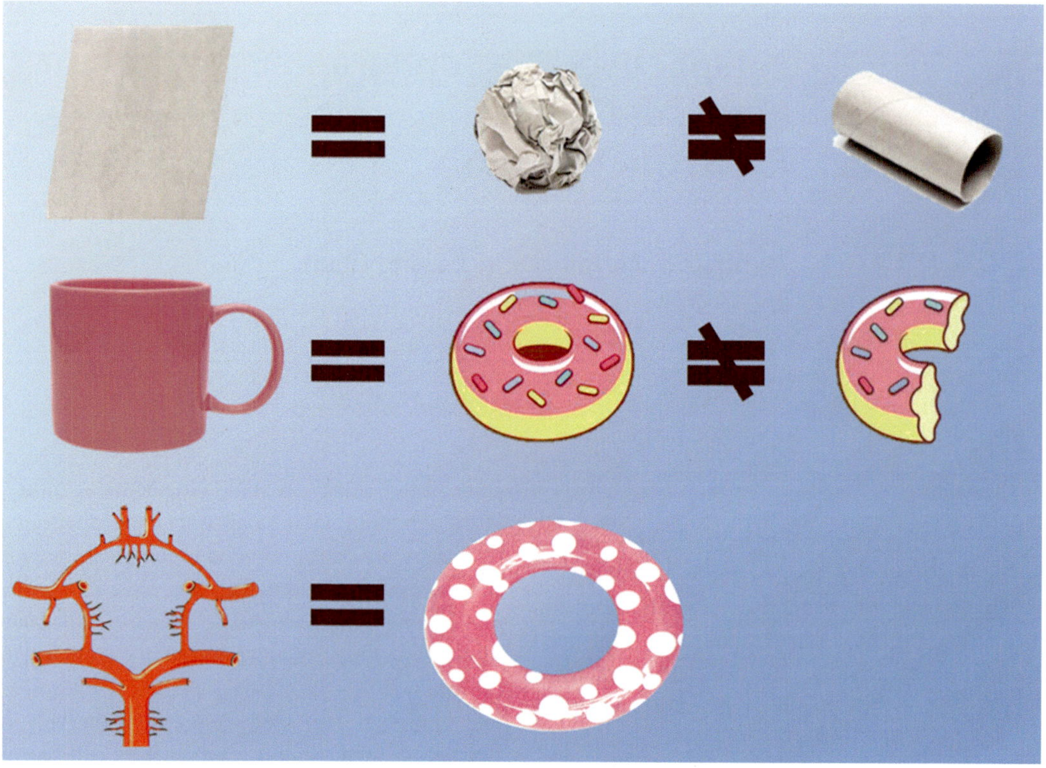

Fig. 13.1 Illustrations for topologically equivalent items. Upper: A twisted piece of paper is topologically equivalent to a flat sheet of paper as long as it is not rolled and glued into a cylinder. Middle: A mug is topologically equivalent to a doughnut, unless a bite has been taken out of the doughnut. It is worth noting that the bite should be large enough to break the circle. Lower: The circle of Willis is topologically equivalent to an inflatable floating ring with holes

13.2 The Application of Topography in the Treatment of Intracranial Aneurysms

We consider some issues that still need to be re-evaluated through extensive clinical experience for intracranial aneurysm surgery, like the homology and heterology among aneurysms and the surgical options' goals and limits. The aneurysms with wide and narrow necks may require different treatment strategies, but they can present with a similar topological structure even with different morphology [1].

The topological structure is evaluated according to the relationship between aneurysms and adjacent arteries. As illustrated in Fig. 13.2a, despite its shape, the aneurysm body can be considered as a bubble, and the perforator(s) and parent artery(s) can be imaged from some holes (necks) on the bubble surface. Therefore, a usual aneurysm with only one narrow neck is equal to a bubble with one hole, but the fusiform or serpentine aneurysms are bubbles with two holes. Although they look different, aneurysms with wide or narrow necks are topologically equivalent. The parent artery's proximal (inflow) or distal (outflow) branches will not affect an aneurysm's topological equivalence (Fig. 13.2b) because they may share a single neck. However, the perforators' appearance can dramatically raise the topological complexity due to their independent necks (Fig. 13.2c). Since there is no limit to a complex aneurysm's topological com-

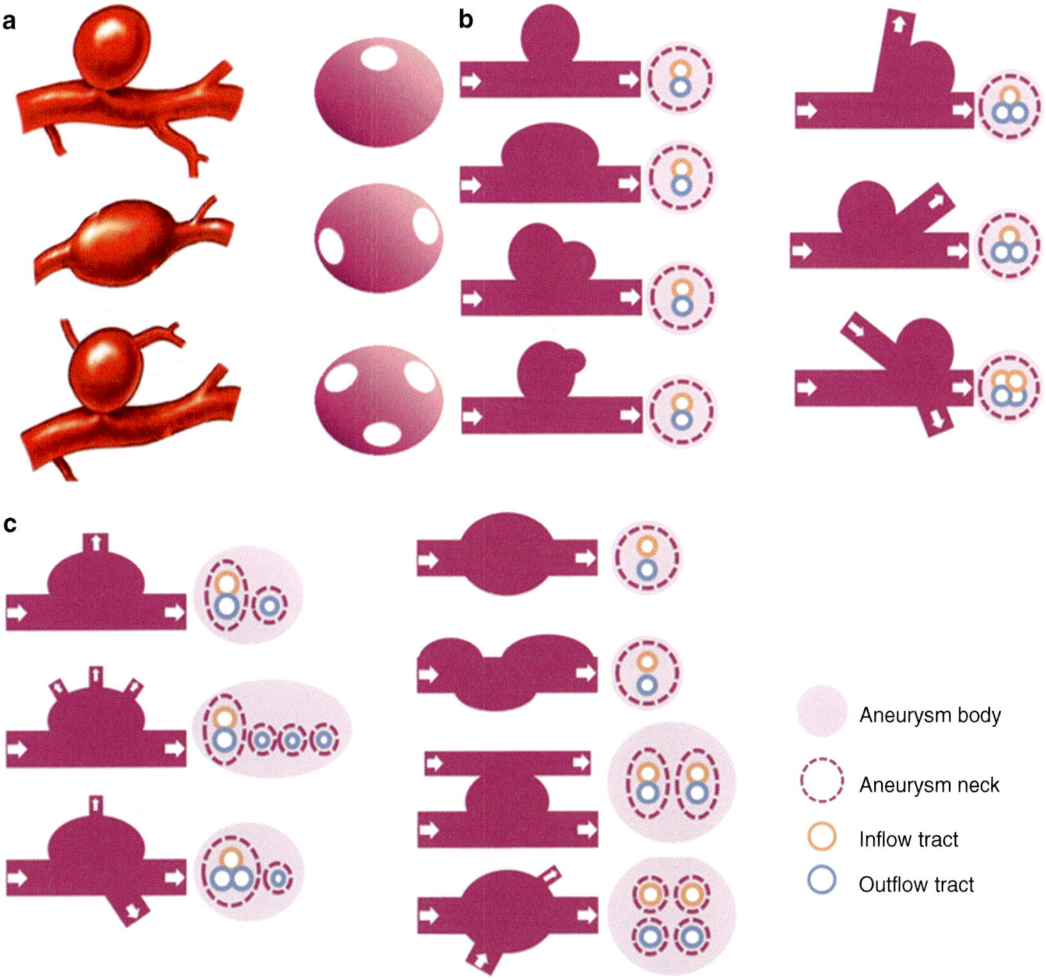

Fig. 13.2 Topology diagrams of aneurysms with various morphologies. (**a**) Topology diagrams of three aneurysm types. (**b**) Various aneurysm morphologies with one neck. (**c**) Some complex aneurysm morphologies with more than one neck (Reproduced from Zou X, Chen L, Mao Y. Commentary: Analysis of Wide-Neck Aneurysms in the Barrow Ruptured Aneurysm Trial. Neurosurgery. 2019; 85(5): E822–24)

plexity, in theory, treating them is oft-sought-after albeit challenging and similar to art.

The intracranial aneurysm treatment concept has shifted over time. Ligation, coiling, or clipping is the concept of simple "isolation," and is mostly taken for granted in treating aneurysms with narrow necks (topologically simple). However, in aneurysms with wide necks, a simple "isolation" approach may become challenging. Nevertheless, when considering topology properties, these aneurysms can theoretically be "isolated" by more complicated "reconstructive" procedures like reconstructive clipping, stent-assisted coiling, or flow diverters regardless of technical difficulty (Fig. 13.3a). When facing topologically complex aneurysms with three or more necks, such simple or reconstructive "isolation" concept does have limitations and becomes inapplicable. Therefore, bypass surgeries may help achieve functional reconstruction instead of structural repair, breaking the topological restrictions (Fig. 13.3b). However, the sufficient dissection of the perforators may not always be easy. Mostly, they will inevitably be occluded during the surgery.

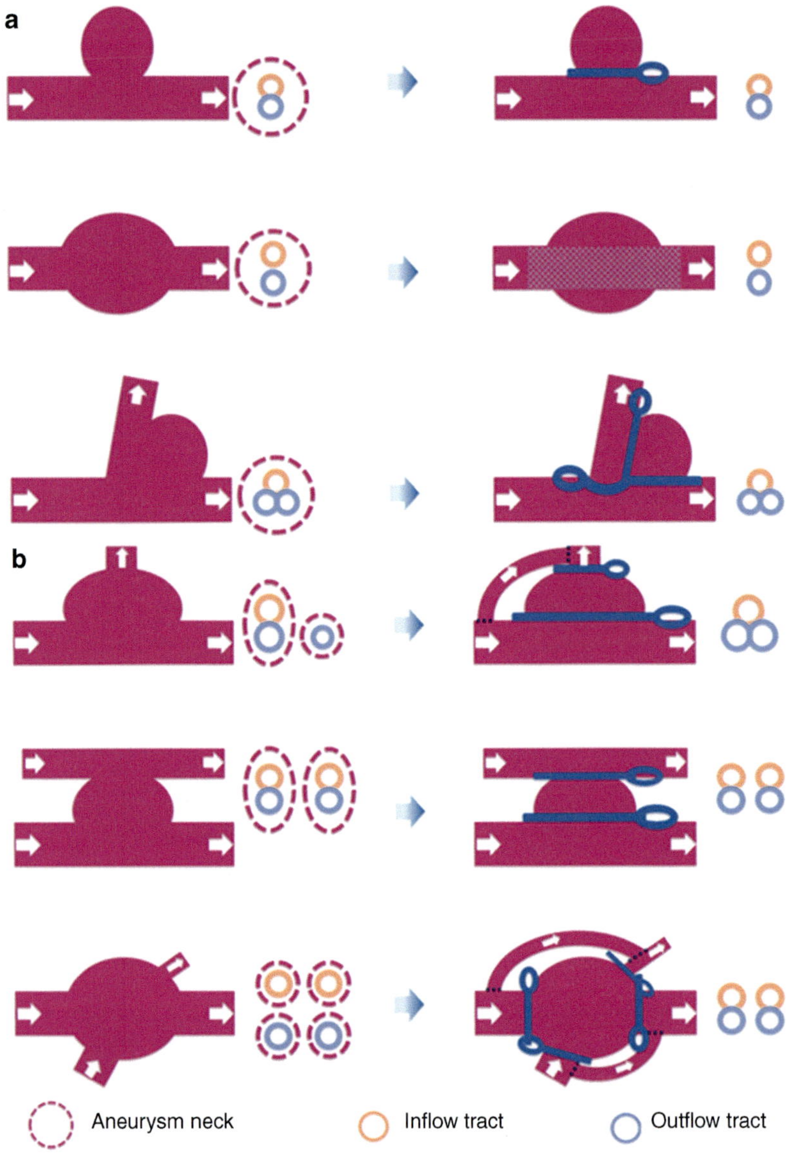

Fig. 13.3 Surgical strategies for aneurysms with different morphologies. (**a**) Surgical options for some topologically simple aneurysms. (**b**) Surgical options for some topologically complex aneurysms (Reproduced from Zou X, Chen L, Mao Y. Commentary: Analysis of Wide-Neck Aneurysms in the Barrow Ruptured Aneurysm Trial. Neurosurgery. 2019; 85(5): E822–24)

Thus, according to the aneurysm's topological complexity, we can propose the following rules of the surgical strategy: (1) Topologically speaking, only the neck encloses the rushing inflow and outflow tracts, and the goal of treatment is to eliminate the neck; (2) aneurysms with one neck have the most simplified topological structure and topological invariance in theory and can be secured by "isolation; (3) although with different morphology, aneurysms with the same topological patterns can be cured with the similar surgical techniques (Fig. 13.4a, b); (4) although with similar morphology, aneurysms with different topological patterns may require different surgical techniques (Fig. 13.4a, c); and (5) each surgical technique has its topological property and restrictions.

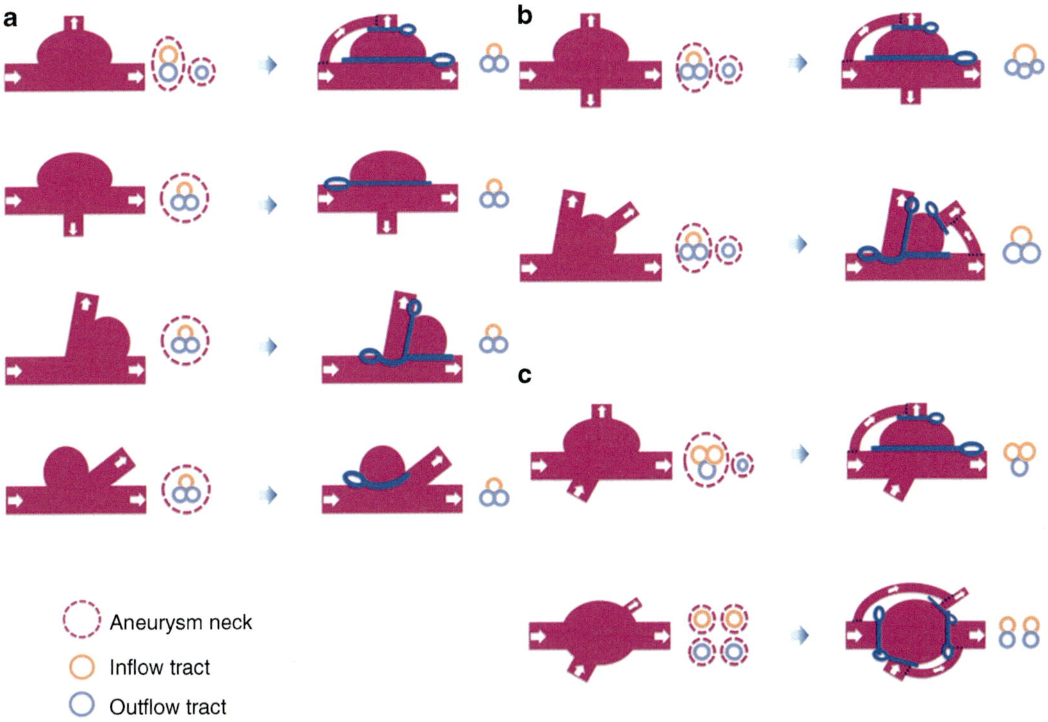

Fig. 13.4 Surgical strategies for aneurysms with various topological types. (**a**) Morphologically similar aneurysms with the same/different topological structure and their similar/different surgery options. (**b**) Morphologically different complex aneurysms with the same topological structure and similar surgical options. (**c**) Morphologically similar complex aneurysms with different topological structures and different surgical options (Reproduced from Zou X, Chen L, Mao Y. Commentary: Analysis of Wide-Neck Aneurysms in the Barrow Ruptured Aneurysm Trial. Neurosurgery. 2019; 85(5): E822–24)

13.3 Topographic Model of Cerebral Revascularization

The optimal surgical strategy selection is influenced by many variables, such as aneurysm morphology, size, vascular architecture, and even the surgeon's preference. However, from the topological perspective, with the "topological neck" enclosing the inflow and/or outflow tract(s) on one side of the aneurysm, different aneurysms may be topologically equivalent, regardless of the abovementioned variables. This enables aneurysms to be categorized into only three basic topological types regarding surgical considerations (Fig. 13.5). Herein, we unify the two basic surgical techniques (clipping and revascularization) and propose the following "grand unification theory" for the surgical treatment of cerebral aneurysms based on their topological types:

Type A: The aneurysms do not incorporate any branches, so their topological neck encloses only one inflow and outflow tract. These aneurysms can be saccular (actually side-wall aneurysms) or nonsaccular (fusiform, dissecting, serpentine, or dolichoectatic aneurysms). This type of aneurysm can be definitively cured by clipping or trapping/resection with flow-replacement revascularization if they are unclippable.

Type B: The aneurysm neck joins the origin of the branches. As there is no real neck on a nonsaccular aneurysm, only bifurcation saccular aneurysms are included in this category. This type of aneurysm is mainly treated by clipping. If direct clipping cannot be achieved, reconstruc-

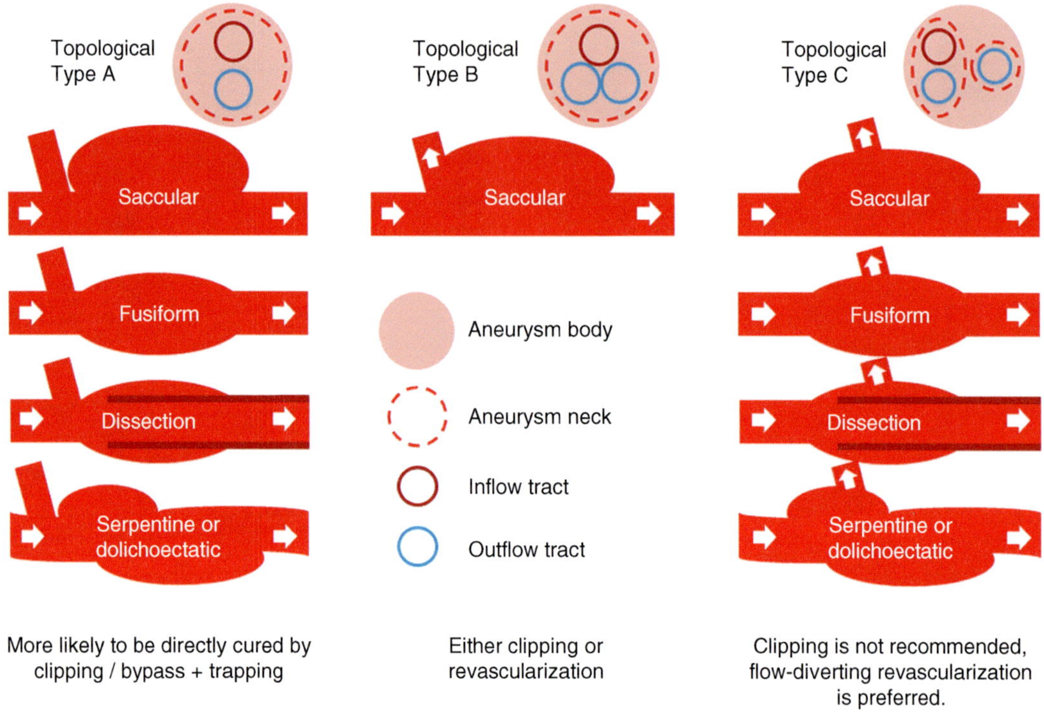

Fig. 13.5 Three basic topological types of cerebral aneurysms

tion techniques or flow-protective/replacement revascularization-assisted clipping/trapping may be applied, requiring the surgeons' maximal creativity.

Type C: Branch(es) arise from the body of the aneurysm. The aneurysm can be saccular or nonsaccular and can have more than one topologic neck. The proximal neck encloses the main inflow and outflow tract(s) of the parent artery, and the distal neck(s) enclose the branching outflow tract(s) only. Revascularization is usually required to eliminate the distal neck(s). Aneurysm trapping/resection with flow-replacement revascularization can be applied when the branch(es) are safe sites for recipient anastomosis. However, if the branches supply a large area, such as perforators, the preferred technique is flow-reversal revascularization combined with proximal occlusion to preserve the perforators' blood flow; distal occlusion has also been recently proposed as an alternative.

Wrapping is the palliative option, and simple parent artery occlusion/aneurysm trapping should be considered the last resort treatment for cerebral aneurysms, which must be performed under close collateral hemodynamic analysis electrophysiological monitoring.

Ultimately, the treatment of intracranial aneurysms is a comprehensive medical procedure. The topological view may provide a more in-depth insight into aneurysms and the limitations of existing surgical procedures. This concise topographic classification system can be considered the basic model for selecting an optimal cerebral aneurysm surgical strategy.

Reference

1. Zou X, Chen L, Mao Y. Commentary: analysis of wide-neck aneurysms in the barrow ruptured aneurysm trial. Neurosurgery. 2019;85(5):E822–4.

Printed by Printforce, the Netherlands